NCLEX-RN Study Guide! Complete Review of NCLEX Examination Concepts

Ultimate Trainer & Test Prep Book To Help Pass The Test!

Author

Kim Nguyen

Table Of Contents

Introduction

The NCLEX stands for "National Council Licensure Examination." It's a test created and developed by the National Council of State Boards of Nursing. In the US, each state has its regulations in terms of how registered nurses are allowed to practice nursing within the state. However, the licensing exam is the same for everyone, and this is known as the NCLEX.

This test is reviewed every three years but in varying timelines. Then the reviewers made the necessary changes to make sure that all of the content of the test remains current. The NCLEX-RN is taken by those who have graduated from registered nursing programs. Applying for this test would cost you around $200. The minimum number of questions for this test is 75 while the maximum number of questions for this test is 265. The other type of NCLEX test is known as the NCLEX-PN, and this is taken by those who have graduated from practical or vocational nursing courses.

Vocational nurses, licensed nurses, and registered nurses can all legally refer to themselves as nurses. That is unlike the other types of healthcare workers who perform the same kinds of tasks. Apart from the type of NCLEX test they take, vocational and licensed nurses differ from registered nurses in terms of the scope of their practice, their education, and the compensation they receive.

What is the NCLEX-RN?

The NCLEX-RN has one main purpose which is to determine whether it's safe for the nurses who take the exam to start their practice as entry-level nurses. This test significantly differs from any other type of test nurses take while they're still studying in nursing school. All exams taken in nursing school are based on the knowledge they learn while they're studying. But the NCLEX-RN tests the analysis and application of the nurses who have already graduated from nursing school. You will get tested on how well you make use of your critical thinking skills in terms of making real-life judgments for nursing-related situations.

The NCLEX-RN framework is based on "Meeting the Client's Needs." This exam has four main categories and eight subcategories, each of which we will discuss in detail later on. The basis of several nursing programs is the medical model wherein students take separate classes namely obstetric, medical, pediatric, surgical, and psychiatric. But when you take the NCLEX-RN, the content from all of these classes are integrated.

Most of the questions on the NCLEX-RN are multiple-choice questions. But there are also other types of questions for you to answer. The one thing that they have in common is that they all contain integrated nursing content. Anyone who takes the NCLEX-RN would have to answer a minimum of 75 questions.

No matter how many questions you're able to answer, you will also have to answer 15 experimental questions which will neither count for you or against you. The purpose of these questions is for the future reference of the administrators of the NCLEX-RN. Although each of the questions doesn't have a time limit, you have up to six hours to finish the whole test, and that includes the tutorial which you will have at the beginning. The exam doesn't involve mandatory breaks, but there are optional breaks you may take during the exam.

Interesting Facts About the NCLEX

The NCLEX-RN is a nationwide exam to license nurses both in Canada and in America. Here are some interesting facts about this test to give you a clearer picture of its purpose and process:

- **The purpose of the NCLEX-RN**

The design of the NCLEX-RN is to evaluate the abilities, skills, and knowledge of the test takers to determine whether they can practice entry-level nursing effectively and safely. It's a type of standardized test utilized by the board of nursing to determine the readiness of the test takers. The owner of the NCLEX-RN (along with the NCLEX-PN) is the National Council of State Boards of Nursing. They're also the ones who develop the exams.

- **Applying for the NCLEX-RN**

Any nurse who has already applied for a nursing license from the state's board of nursing can register to take the NCLEX-RN. The state board is responsible for determining every applicant's eligibility to take the test. Each state has its guidelines and requirements for determining eligibility.

Once the state board has verified the applicant's eligibility, he will receive an Authorization to Take the Test or an ATT. The applicant will also receive a list of all the possible testing centers along with the steps to take when scheduling an appointment to take the test. After registration for the NCLEX-RN is created, it remains open for a whole year waiting for applicant eligibility. Those who receive an ATT must take the test within the dates written on their ATT.

- **Who is the NCLEX-RN for**

The NCLEX-RN is a test for those who have graduated with a Bachelor's Degree in Nursing or an Associate's Degree in Nursing. The exam utilizes a five-step nursing process wherein each of the questions falls into one of these five steps namely assessment, evaluation, diagnosis, implementation, and planning.

- **There are various patterns and types of NCLEX-RN questions**

The design of the NCLEX-RN uses the Computerized Adaptive Testing or CAT format. About 90% of these questions are multiple-choice. The remaining questions are of different types which we will be discussed more later on. One thing's for sure: with all of the questions included in the NCLEX-RN, none of them are repeated.

- **The NCLEX-RN scoring is quite complicated**

The NCLEX-RN covers a wide-range of nursing-related material. The scoring of this examination is based on critical thinking. The exam has a computational algorithm which assesses the correctness of the answers within the context of their difficulty and topic knowledge. The grading is done by comparing the answers to pre-established standards. Those who either meet or exceed those standards pass the NCLEX-RN while those who don't, fail.

There's no standard percentage or number of questions needed to pass the NCLEX-RN. This is because each of the questions would depend on how you answered the previous questions. Therefore, you may receive between 75 – 265 questions depending on how well you do on the test. The computer will randomly and continuously generate questions for you from each of the categories until you've met all of the test plan requirements.

- **The NCLEX-RN begins with the preparation**

The NCLEX-RN isn't just some random test that you would take when you want to. Even if you earn straight A's throughout nursing school, this doesn't mean that you will pass the NCLEX-RN. For this test, you should spend at least a month or two studying for the test. Think about it, each time you try to take the test, you would have to spend $200! So you might as well prepare well before taking it to ensure that you get a good result. From reviewing the right materials to taking practice tests, and more, there are plenty of steps you can take to prepare for the NCLEX-RN before taking it.

- **Finding out the results of the NCLEX-RN**

After you've taken the NCLEX-RN, the next step is to wait until the results come out. The official test results get posted on the board of nursing or the regulatory body's website. Also, they will send the results to you by mail. If the board of nursing in your state is part of the Quick Results Service, then you may receive your results (although unofficial) after two business days for a fee.

- **Unfortunately, some people don't pass the NCLEX-RN**

This is a sad fact that's true for any other type of exam. After all, if everybody passes the exam each time, it must be too easy! The good news is that you can re-take the NCLEX-RN after a waiting period of 45 days if you didn't pass on your first attempt.

FAQs about the NCLEX-RN

For nursing students to get a nursing license, they must first pass the NCLEX-RN. In other words, this test stands between all of the nursing graduates and their ability to become a licensed nurse to practice their craft. Even if you don't pass on your first attempt, you can retake the exam. Of course, any nurse would prefer to pass the exam on the first try. Let's answer some of the most common questions about the NCLEX-RN to help you understand it better:

1. What is tested on the NCLEX-RN?

The National Council Licensure Examination or the NCLEX-RN is a test which determines your readiness to start practicing as an entry-level nurse. Unlike the knowledge-based exams which you have taken frequently in nursing school, the NCLEX-RN tests your critical thinking skills in terms of how you make nursing judgments. Therefore, you must make yourself as familiar as possible with the test, especially if you want to perform well on it.

2. What is the NCLEX-RN test plan?

This is an outline of the NCLEX-RN. You can think of the test plan as a "blueprint" by the National Council of State Boards of Nursing. It's important to understand this test plan and how it works when you're preparing to take the test. All of the information about test plans and the NCLEX-RN for both educators and candidates through the National Council of State Boards of Nursing.

3. How can you prepare for the NCLEX-RN?

There are several ways for you to prepare for the NCLEX-RN. You can find reliable review materials to help you. Also, you can either obtain a test plan or build one for yourself and use it along with your review materials. Another way to prepare for the test is to take practice tests or download some test questions and practice answering those. Such efforts will go a long way in terms of your preparedness for when you need to take the NCLEX-RN.

4. What is the passing standard for the NCLEX-RN?

Every three years, the National Council of State Boards of Nursing Board of Directors review the test, the test plan, and the passing standards. They do this so they can make the necessary changes to comply with any changes made in terms of the field of nursing as well as the competence requirements of entry-level nurses. From now until the March 21, 2019, the passing standard for the NCLEX-RN is 0.00 logits.

5. How are the questions distributed on the NCLEX-RN?

Most of the time, nursing students focus on the distribution of questions when taking exams. The same thing goes for the NCLEX-RN. Here is a breakdown of the distribution of questions on this test:

- Health Promotion and Maintenance – 9%

- Psychosocial Integrity – 9%

- Basic Care and Comfort – 9%

- Safety and Infection Control – 12%

- Reduction of Risk Potential – 12%

- Physiological Adaptation – 14%

- Pharmacological and Parenteral Therapies – 15%

- Management of Care – 20%

Ultimately, the format of the NCLEX-RN is made according to the needs of the candidates. This means that it includes modifications in the test's length. The percentages of the question distribution may also be different from one candidate to another.

The bottom line is this, even if there are any changes made to the NCLEX-RN, you don't need to concern yourself with them. You may want to learn about those changes (which we will discuss later on), but it won't affect how you should prepare. Just by taking extra time and effort to learn more about the NCLEX-RN, you're already placing yourself ahead of the curve!

6. How many times can you take the NCLEX-RN?

Unfortunately, some people don't pass the NCLEX-RN. After all, it's designed to determine the readiness of everyone who takes the test. So if you happen to fail the NCLEX-RN, this means that you need to prepare more for it. The good news is that you can retake the test after 45 days.

Also, you're allowed to take the NCLEX-RN up to eight times a year. When you think about it, that's a lot of times to retake the test! This is why it's important to prepare as much as you can from the first time you take the NCLEX-RN.

7. What score should you aim to pass the NCLEX-RN?

There's no specific number of questions you must answer correctly to pass this test. The algorithm of the NCLEX-RN considers the questions' difficulty and the variety of topics which they cover. The test will end when you've run into one of these scenarios:

- When the adaptive testing determines that you've sufficiently passed each of the subject areas of the exam;

- When you've reached the maximum number of hours allowed for the test; or

- When you've answered the maximum number of questions.

Chapter 1: Preparing for the NCLEX-RN Exam

Every nursing graduate who aspires to become a registered nurse must take the NCLEX-RN. This test is designed to assess the knowledge, skills, and abilities of nursing graduates to ensure that they are ready to work as an entry-level nurse. So if you're planning to take this test, you must prepare well to increase your chances of passing on your first try.

All About the NCLEX-RN Exam

The nursing profession is both a science and an art which is founded on a professional body of knowledge which incorporates concepts from psychological, biological, social, and physical sciences along with the liberal arts. Nursing professionals learn about the human condition across the entire lifespan along with the relationship of people with others and with their environment. Nursing is a very dynamic discipline which continues to evolve and which requires critical thinking to use skills, technologies, and knowledge which are becoming increasingly complex. The goal of this profession is to prevent any potential complications and illnesses; to promote, protect, facilitate, and restore comfort; encourage health; and provide dignity in dying.

The NCLEX-RN is a computerized adaptive test with a variable length. It doesn't come in the form of oral or paper-and-pencil examinations. You will be given up to 6 hours to complete the test including all of the following:

- · An instructional tutorial about the NCLEX-RN.

- · Two optional breaks which have been pre-programmed which you may or may not take. You will be alerted by the computer when it's time to take these breaks.

- · Other breaks which you want to take.

- · The NCLEX-RN itself.

After answering the minimum number of

questions and based on how well you've answered them, the NCLEX-RN will stop if you're either below or above the standard for passing. Putting it simply, the NCLEX-RN stops once you've passed or when it's certain that you've failed. Also, the test stops after you've answered the maximum number of questions or when you've reached the 6-hour time limit.

During the test, the computer screen will only show you one question at a time. You can take as long as you want to answer the question on the screen, but you can't move on to the next question until you've answered it. This means that even if you're uncertain, you must answer the given question if you want to proceed to the next ones. Rather than guessing the answer, try to think about the question and give the best answer you can think of. Keep a steady pace so you won't be rushing when you realize that the time limit is fast-approaching.

Types of Exam Questions

Part of preparing for the NCLEX-RN is to know the types of questions to expect. Knowing the types of questions gives you more confidence in taking the test. And if you've reviewed all of the concepts well, you might be able to breeze through the entire NCLEX-RN and pass it on your first try (after all, it thinking positive never hurts)! To help you out, here are the types of exam questions to expect on the NCLEX-RN:

- **Exhibit or Chart**

For these types of questions, you would have to evaluate an exhibit or chart then answer the questions which will be presented. If you've had tests where you used pie charts or bar graphs to select the correct answer, then you would be familiar with how to answer these types of questions.

- **Fill in the Blanks**

These types of questions don't mean that you have to provide essays or short answers. In the NCLEX-RN, fill in the blanks questions are for performing calculations. You would have to calculate the drip rate for administering an IV fluid or the dosage of the medication to administer to a patient. Then you would record your answer on the blank. You will be given specific instructions on rounding so that you can give your best answer.

- **Graphic or Audio**

For graphic questions, you would be presented with a question or scenario, and you must choose the correct answer by selecting the correct graphic. For audio questions, you would listen to a short recording then choose the correct answer based on the question or scenario you've heard.

- **Hot Spot**

These types of questions would require you to identify the areas on graphics or pictures. For instance, you may be asked to highlight the parts of the chest where you would assess the sounds of the heart. You will be tasked to identify the "hot spot" based on the question that is asked.

- **Multiple Response or Multiple Choice**

These types of questions are very common in different types of exams in different subjects. You may have been answering multiple choice questions since you were in kindergarten! For this type, you will be given a scenario or a question and a list of possible answers. Then all you have to do is select the correct or the best answer from the list.

- **Order Response**

These types of questions would ask you to place selections in the correct order. You may be given different types of patient situations wherein you would have to demonstrate the correct management of care. Or you may have a scenario wherein a patient comes in, and you would have to arrange the steps according to what you would do first, second, third, and so on.

Apart from knowing the types of questions, you will answer on the NCLEX-RN, it's also helpful to know all about the questions themselves. To do this, let's break down the structure of the questions. Each question has:

- an **item** which is the whole question and the answer

- a **stem** which is the actual question or what you are being asked

For the stem, this has a couple of characteristics for you to think about namely:

- **Complete sentence**

- **Incomplete sentence,** which becomes complete when you supply the correct answer

- **Negative** which asks a question about

what is false

- **Positive** which asks a question about what is true

The Steps to Follow for the NCLEX-RN Exam

If you're planning to take the NCLEX-RN, there are certain steps you need to take even before you take the test. Here is a quick rundown of these steps for your reference:

1. Visit the board of nursing in your territory or state and apply for licensure. They will provide you with a list of requirements you have to prepare.

2. Register for the NCLEX-RN online, by telephone or by mail.

   a) Make sure to use your complete, legal name upon registration which matches the name on the ID you will present at the testing center.

   b) If you register for the NCLEX-RN through email, all of your subsequent communication will be done through email.

c) All registrations for the NCLEX-RN will stay open for a specific period (365 days). During this time, the board of nursing will determine whether you're eligible to take the test or not.

d) After paying the $200 registration fee for the NCLEX-RN, you won't be able to refund it no matter what your reason is.

3. Receive the confirmation of your registration.

4. Receive eligibility from the board of nursing in your territory or state.

5. Receive the Authorization to Test or ATT. If you have not received this after two weeks from the date you received your confirmation, you may contact the board of nursing.

   a. The ATT contains validity dates, and you should take the NCLEX-RN within those dates.
   b. The name on your ID must match with the name on your ATT exactly.

6. Schedule your NCLEX-RN appointment either online or by telephone.

7. Show up early on your test date and time then take the test!

Practical Tips for Taking the NCLEX-RN Exam for the First Time

After you've graduated from nursing school, you will feel great about yourself and for a good reason! Graduating from this course is a huge accomplishment in itself. But your work isn't over. For you to become a registered nurse, you must take the NCLEX-RN and pass the test. Apart from reviewing all of the concepts, here are some practical tips for you to consider:

1. Understand the NCLEX-RN

You must learn all that you can about the exam. From what it is, the format, the structure, the types of questions, and more, there's a lot for you to learn!

2. Learn stress management

Although preparing for the test can be very stressful, you must learn how to manage your stress. That way, you can focus more on your studying than on your apprehensions.

3. Know your own learning or study style

We all have our learning or study style and knowing yours will allow you to tailor your study plan according to your strengths which, in turn, will make it more effective.

4. Create a study plan

Preparing for the NCLEX-RN requires a lot of work and organization. By creating your study plan, you will have a better idea of everything you need to cover and how you will be able to study everything.

5. Don't just draw from your experiences

If you have tried working in healthcare facilities (like as part of your schooling or as a sideline), don't let those experiences cloud your thinking. You still need to study and prepare to ensure that you will do well on the NCLEX-RN.

6. Improve your test-taking skills

To do this, you must also learn some test-taking strategies such as learning how to eliminate the wrong answers, avoiding the answers which offer "extremes," and others.

7. Invest in the right resources

These include purchasing review books (such as this one!), practice exam books or even enrolling yourself in a review course specifically for the NCLEX-RN.

8. Try answering practice questions or practice tests

There are plenty of practice questions and practice tests available online. You can also purchase books which include these questions which are similar to those which you will have to answer on the NCLEX-RN. Take advantage of all these so you can get all the practice you need.

9. Join a study group

A lot of people find that learning with others and having discussions while studying is more effective than just learning on their own. If you're one of these people, you may want to join a study group as part of your preparation.

10. Believe in your own abilities

Finally, you must believe in your abilities! There's no point in taking the exam if you don't think you can pass it. After you've studied and prepared for it, try your best when you take the exam and hope for the best!

Understanding the NCLEX-RN Test Plan

The NCLEX-RN test plan is a tool which you can use to prepare for the test. This plan is organized systematically under broad categories. Some of these categories have their subcategories which are also broken down into detailed activity statements. The contents of this test plan are divided into eight major categories. Then the NCSBN develops a range of percentages that each of these categories will appear on the exam.

There are specifically integrated processes which are important to nursing practice, and all of these are incorporated throughout the main categories. These processes include:

- **Caring**, which is the interaction between the nurse and patient in an environment of mutual trust and respect.

- **Documentation and communication**, which includes the

non-verbal and verbal interactions between the nurse and the patient as well as the significant others of the patient and the other members of the patient's healthcare team.

- **The nursing process**, which is the clinical reasoning and scientific approach to patient care.

- **Spirituality and culture**, which is the interaction of the nurse and the patient which considers and recognizes the individual preferences to patient care.

- **Teaching and learning**, which is facilitating the acquisition of attitudes, skills, and knowledge to promote a good change in behavior.

Familiarizing yourself with and using the NCLEX-RN test plan will help you prepare for the test more adequately. By using this as your study tool, you will be able to focus on the most important information to study to be able to answer the questions on the test in the best possible way. So now, let's go through the different categories of the NCLEX-RN to help you prepare.

Chapter 2: Category Review Guide for Basic Care and Comfort

To maintain a patient's physiological integrity, the first thing you must do is to take a basic evaluation of all the patients. This step involves collecting information which will help you determine what kind of care the patients need. This is where Basic Care and Comfort comes in.

Patients who are either semi-ambulatory or non-ambulatory might need some help in terms of positioning to prevent the formation of ulcers. Of course, non-ambulatory patients need more time and effort from you, especially in terms of helping them with their personal hygiene. It's important to maintain the cleanliness of such patients, especially those who are incontinent.

As a nurse, your job is to respect all of the wishes of your patients. For instance, if they prefer alternative therapy, you may have to assist them in terms of working through their pain according to their individual preferences and needs. Because of this, it's important to make yourself aware of the alternative methods to pain management otherwise known as non-pharmacological comfort interventions. For instance, instead of taking pharmaceuticals, some patients might prefer deep breathing techniques, meditation, herbal remedies, and the like.

Keep in mind that being sick is extremely draining. And the difficult part is that a lot of patients don't understand why they don't feel better right away after just taking a single dose of antibiotics. Rest, sleep, and proper education will help your patients understand the process of recovery which is not an instantaneous thing. For this category, it's important to learn everything you can to be able to take care of your patients in the best possible way.

The Basic Concepts Covered in Basic Care and Comfort

This category contains all of the information you may need to provide basic care and comfort to your patients. This means that you need to assist your patients to perform their daily activities. In the NCLEX-RN, this category accounts for about 9% of the questions:

Assistive Devices

This aspect of the category includes:

- evaluating the patient's utilization of assistive devices;

- managing the care of a patient who utilizes prosthetic apparatuses or assistive devices;

- improving the patient's ability to overcome his/her sensory or physical impairment; and

- evaluating the proper utilization of the assistive devices by the patient.

There are different types of assistive devices which can be utilized by patients depending on their impairment:

- Assistive devices for patients with hearing difficulties include sound amplifiers, hearing aids, and other types of alerting devices.

- Assistive devices for physical safety and ambulation include crutches, canes, and walkers.

- Options for people who are visually impaired or those who have vision deficits include walking canes, Braille devices or even a service animal.

- For patients who suffer from speech impairments (such as those who suffered from a stroke) might need picture boards, word boards or even handheld electronic devices which generate speed. Such patients may need these devices so that they can communicate properly.

Each patient required a complete evaluation. And as a nurse, your job is to perform these evaluations to determine the right type of assistive device which will be most appropriate for your patients. Even though two patients suffer from the same impairment or condition, they may require different devices and therapies for their optimal functioning and health.

This means that no two patients who suffer from communication, auditory, speech or physical deficits may require the same type of assistive devices. Therefore, it's important for you to individualize your recommendations based on the individual needs of your patients.

After completing the evaluation and determining the best time of assistive devices to use on your patients, the next thing to do is to educate your patients on how to use these devices. You must make sure that your patients will be able to use their assistive devices safely. Also, you must make sure that your patients will be able to safely and efficiently perform their daily activities while using the assistive devices recommended for them. You must also allow your patients the maximum amount of independence as possible to prepare them for when you need to leave them on their own.

Finally, you must also evaluate how well your patients can use their own assistive devices. The best way for you to evaluate this is by observing how your patients use the said devices. Proper usage means that your patients can utilize the devices effectively and safely without causing injuries to themselves. If not, you can either keep on training your patient or think about assigning a different type of device to use.

Elimination

Elimination is the next part of this category, and it's important for all patients. As a nurse, it's your job to evaluate and manage patients who are experiencing a change in their urinary or bowel elimination. For this section, you also have to perform tasks such as:

- skin care for the incontinent patients;

- irrigations of the ears, eyes, bladder, and more;

- alternative measures to encourage a patient's toileting or voiding schedule;

- evaluating your patient's elimination ability, especially if this is either restored or maintained; and

- recording outputs.

Helping your patients meet their elimination needs is crucial. Both the bladder and bowel function may change. This means that you need to provide the proper nursing interventions for the well-being and health of your patients.

There are several reasons why a patient might develop a change in his bladder or bowel functions. These reasons include but aren't limited to:

- age;

- a decrease in muscular tone;

- medication use;

- neurological disorders;

- physical disorders; and

- psychological issues.

Therefore, you need to make a full evaluation of your patient to determine the proper interventions to perform.

Urinary elimination which is also known as micturition is a natural bodily process which may come with a lot of issues the most common of which is UTI. Here are some of the most common terms relating to this condition and other urinary issues:

- **Anuria**, which is a lack of or a very minimal amount of urine production.

- **Oliguria**, which is a urine output that's less than normal.

- **Polyuria**, which is an excessive urine production.

- **Dysuria**, which is difficult or painful urination.

- **Urgency**, which is the uncontrollable, strong, and sudden urge to urinate.

- **Urinary incontinence**, which is the loss of bladder control or involuntary urine leakage.

- **Urinary retention**, which is the buildup of urine in the patient's bladder because he can't empty it completely.

The other type of elimination known as defecation is the passage of stool. To identify the problems your patient suffers from in terms of defecation, you need to perform an evaluation based on your patient's health and age. Here are the most common terms which are related to bowel issues:

- **Constipation** which means that the patient has only three bowel movements or less each week.

- **Diarrhea** which means that the patient is eliminating loose or watery stool.

- **Fecal impaction** which means that your patient isn't able to pass stool because it has already accumulated inside his rectum and has become rock-hard.

- **Flatulence** which is the frequent expulsion of GI gas.

There are times when you will have to perform irrigations of your patient's bodily orifices. This is essential as a type of therapeutic intervention to maintain the proper functioning of your patient's organs. The irrigations to perform may include ear, eye, bladder, colostomy (fecal diversion), and urostomy (urinary diversion). For colostomy, you must use the clean technique. For all the other types, you must use the sterile technique.

For any incontinent patient, you must provide careful and constant skin care. You must always wash and dry any skin that's exposed to feces and urine. Also, using specific types of barrier products such as skin sealants, moisture barrier ointments or pastes, and solid skin barriers help prevent skin complications and breakdown.

Non-ambulatory patients or those who aren't able to urinate may require a urinary catheter. You must use the sterile technique during catheter insertion because this procedure has a high risk of infection.

Successfully managing bladder and bowel issues means that your patients are already able to empty their stool and urine regularly, painlessly, and without urgency. For some patients, they may have to undergo bowel or bladder training to have better control over their elimination.

Mobility and Immobility

As a nurse, you must be able to:

- assess your patient's range of mobility, motion, strength, motor skills, and gait;

- recognize any complications of immobility;

- use your know-how of psychomotor skills when you provide care to your immobile clients;

- evaluate the skin health of your patient and initiate the required measures to prevent the breakdown of the skin or maintain the integrity of the skin;

- assess the patient's response to the interventions meant to minimize the complications of immobility; and

- execute the required interventions to improve circulation.

The mobility of patients is crucial to their psychological and physical health. Mobility means that the patients CAN move purposefully, easily, and freely in their environment. This is essential for their daily lives, overall health, and recovery. Therefore, you must evaluate any mobility deficiencies which may be corrected with the proper interventions which you will implement into your patients' care plans.

The best way to assess the mobility (or immobility) of your patient is through direct visualization. You may also use standardized tests during your assessment. However, simply observing how your patients sit, stand, move around, walk, and such can provide you with good information about their abilities. If you discover any deficiencies, one intervention you may employ is the use of assistive devices which we have already discussed.

Completely immobile patients, especially those who are on complete bed rest are at-risk for life-threatening complications both psychological and physical. Therefore, you must familiarize yourself with all of the possible adverse effects of immobility and the intervention options you may take. The most common immobility causes include:

- impairment of the motor system;

- impairment of the nervous system;

- medications;

- pain;

- psychological issues; and

- weakness.

The adverse effects of immobility may affect a patient's:

- **Musculoskeletal system**

When a patient isn't able to move this system of his body, this may lead to weakness, muscle atrophy, calcium-loss from the skeletal system, and more. To avoid these complications, you must implement exercises which improve your patient's range of motion along with muscular exercises which the patient can do in bed. You can even make use of a tilt table to stimulate weight-bearing exercises in some patients.

- **Respiratory system**

To maintain the health of the patient's respiratory system and prevent complications, you need to implement inspiratory exercises such as incentive spirometry, deep breathing, and more. Also, some patients may need postural percussion, vibration, and drainage to mobilize their secretions.

- **Skin**

Completely immobile patients have a high risk of skin breakdown. To prevent this, frequent repositioning is essential. Also, remember that the nutritional and fluid needs of patients are crucial to the health of their skin. Other interventions may include the use of assistive and supportive devices to prevent the breakdown of skin and the formation of ulcerations.

- **Venous circulatory system**

Here, the muscular contractions increase the venous blood flow coming from the lower extremities to the heart and lungs which may cause some complications. To encourage proper circulation, you may use anti-embolic devices. Apart from this, you must also implement motion exercises which are either passive, active or active-assisted. Also, implement frequent repositioning and positioning along with mobilization and routine exercises, rehabilitative exercises, and occupational or physical therapy.

- **Others**

The other types of physiologic changes a patient might experience because of immobility are weight gain, bowel alterations, urinary complications, psychological issues, and electrolyte imbalances.

To promote the correct body alignment of immobile patients, you need to perform special positioning. This will also help maintain the proper physiological functioning. Therefore, you must familiarize yourself with the assistive devices and positions needed to maintain proper positioning. Also, make sure to educate your patients on the importance of proper body alignment and positioning and how he/she can help with the process.

Some patients may need the utilization of traction devices both to achieve and to maintain the proper position for their healing. These are commonly used for patients who have suffered a fracture, but they can also be used for other types of serious medical conditions. As a nurse, you're responsible for setting up the device, maintaining it, and ensuring the proper positioning as well as the comfort of the patient. Also, you may have to make adjustments to the device as needed.

When it comes to mobility, it's your job as a nurse to determine whether or not your patients are meeting the goals expected of them. There are other types of interventions which you may use along with the ones we have discussed to ensure the health, safety, and the recovery of your patients.

Non-Pharmacological Comfort Interventions

In this section, you will evaluate the patient's need for:

- alternative medicine;

- complementary medicine;

- non-curative treatments;

- palliative care;

- symptom management; and

- other types of appropriate therapies.

You must evaluate the pain level of your patients as well and apply your knowledge of pathophysiology to the interventions of comfort care. You must be able to effectively integrate complementary and alternative therapies into your patients' care plans. Often, the measures needed for patient comfort involve the utilization of non-pharmacological interventions. Again, different patients require different interventions so you must be able to determine which ones are right for your patients.

The interventions to employ would depend on your assessment of the patient. Depending on the individual preferences and needs of your patients, some of them may be more suited to traditional therapies such as homeopathy, massage, dietary supplements, and more.

Pain is an important part of this section, and this sensation is highly subjective, individualized, and complex. You must familiarize yourself with the theories about the phenomenon of pain along with the phases and types of pain. The proper management of pain starts with the evaluation of your patient's care plan. Asking your patient to give a subjective description of the pain is the most dependable indicator. For adults, you can use facial or numeric pain scales. But for children below three years of age, you may use standardized or behavioral scales for pain assessments.

There several alternative therapies which may have a positive effect on the overall mood of your patient. These include relaxation sounds, low lighting, warm blankets, and more. Simple as these measures are, they can increase your patient's overall sense of well-being and security. You must also know the contraindications to these alternative therapies. Depending on your patient's medication regimen, condition or diagnosis, some therapies might not be safe or appropriate.

When it comes to palliative care, nurses play a huge role and most of the time, you would serve as the coordinator for this type of care. The most important parts of palliative care are family support, pain control, and symptom management. Also, you must have frequent conversations about the goals of your patient in terms of end-of-life support along with executing the required intervention. Your main focus here is the patient's spiritual, emotional, physical, and psychosocial needs.

When a patient is near-death, he/she

experiences several emotional, psychological, and physical changes. During this difficult time, you must take care of your patients and their families as well. When you're assisting your patients, you need to focus on their comfort. Also, your interventions must be based on the individual needs of your patient. The main goal is for your patient to be free of pain.

Nurses also play an important role in helping the patient's family members understand what the patient is going through. It's also important to help them accept any changes they will see in the patient as he/she is nearing the end of his/her life. There is a need to educate and counsel the patients as well as their loved ones to make the process as comfortable and pain-free as possible.

As you're assessing the outcome of any comfort measures and alternative therapies, you must ask for the feedback of your patient and incorporate this into your assessment. Apart from verbal feedback, you must also observe any non-verbal behavior and body posturing of your patient. Also, consider the stated goals of your patients to ensure that you're meeting all of their emotional, spiritual, and physical needs.

Nutrition and Oral Hydration

In this section, you'll learn the importance of oral hydration and nutrition in nursing care. To take care of your patients, you must be able to evaluate your patients' ability to eat properly and to look for any actual or potential interactions between the medications they're taking and the food they're eating. As a nurse, it's your responsibility to:

- assess the side effects of the tube feeding then intervene if needed;

- deliver your patient's nutrition via intermittent or continuous tube feeding; and

- monitor your patient's intake, output, and hydration status then intervene accordingly.

One of the most important priorities of nurses is to promote the overall health and wellness of the patients. To do this, you must make sure that your patients have the proper intake of water along with the vitamins, minerals, and nutrients which come from the food they eat. To do this, you must have a working knowledge of the major food groups along with all of your patients' needs based on their condition, weight, age, and their ability to drink and eat by themselves.

You must perform a nutritional assessment of all your patients. Only after you do this will you be able to assess the real condition of your patients and determine whether they have deficiencies or not. Then, you can start working on the following:

- **Calorie counts**

Counting calories involves calculating the number of grams of carbohydrates, protein, and fat consumed by your patients. You can perform the calculations yourself and educate your patients on how to do this as well.

- **Food restrictions**

Apart from the restrictions from the health conditions of patients, some may also have restrictions because of medication interactions or allergies. You must be aware of all these restrictions if you want to effectively take care of the nutrition and oral hydration of your patients.

- **Managing the intake of food**

It's also your responsibility to help your

patients lose, gain or maintain their current weight. To do this, you must come up with a dietary plan which meets the needs of your patients based on your evaluation. Make sure to create a healthy and balanced diet plan which includes different types of foods.

- **Mathematical calculations**

You may also have to perform some mathematical calculations with regards to the hydration and nutrition of your patients. Some examples of calculations are BMI, calorie counts, and others.

- **Nutritional requirements**

Although patients who don't suffer from serious conditions may only need to follow a well-rounded and balanced diet, some of your patients might suffer from specific health conditions which means that they have specific diet restrictions. In such cases, you must be able to help them achieve all of their nutritional requirements despite these restrictions.

- **Patient preferences**

Often, patients have their preferences in terms of the types of food and how much food or water they take. It's important to speak to your patients about these preferences as you're developing their nutritional care plan.

- **Physical ability**

For your patients to have the proper hydration and oral nutrition, they must be able to eat by themselves, chew well, and swallow without choking. You must also check their dentition as this may have an impact on their physical ability to consume properly. Other factors which may affect this ability include side effects caused by therapies or even neurological conditions.

- **Supplements**

For some patients, they may need to take specific nutritional supplements along with their diets. In such a case, you may have to recommend the proper supplements to your patients based on what they need.

As much as possible, you must encourage your patients to eat on their own. Although it's your job to help them consume all that they need to, your ultimate goal is to allow your patients to do the task independently. If your patients require assistive devices to do this, you must include these in their care plan.

If your patients aren't able to eat independently or they're not able to get sufficient amounts of food orally, you may give them enteral nutrition. You may give this type of nutrition in bolus form, intermittently or continuously. For this procedure, you must carefully maintain the ostomy sites as well as the tubes in terms of their cleanliness and proper positioning. This is important to ensure patency and optimal functioning.

Another important part of this section is the monitoring of your patients' intake and output every day. Careful monitoring is crucial for proper care and management. The results you obtain from your monitoring can be helpful in explaining any changes in your patients such as their weight, vital signs, hydration status, and laboratory values.

In terms of hydration, there are two main categories of fluid imbalances which may occur in patients. The first is dehydration or a fluid deficit and second is edema or an excess of fluids. Each of these categories has its clinical features as well as the corresponding changes which occur in the patients. There are several factors which may cause the fluid imbalances including medications, gender, age, underlying medical conditions, and more.

Personal Hygiene

In this section, you will have to assess your patients in terms of their personal hygiene habits. It's your job to determine the routines of your patients and if these routines are sufficient. Otherwise, you may have to intervene or educate your patients with regards to the essential adaptation for their daily living activities. Personal hygiene is an important part of life. Therefore, you must also be able to help your patients with this.

Just like any other procedure, assessment is the first step. As you evaluate your patients, make sure to check their ability to:

- shave;

- shower or bathe;

- perform perineal, hair, nail, and foot care;

- perform proper denture care;

- perform proper mouth and oral care; and

- wash their hands properly.

Your patients will require varying levels of

nursing intervention and care depending on their individual needs. As you're evaluating your patients, make sure to identify the areas which need intervention and education. For some patients, you may have to incorporate special tools and assistive devices to help them with their personal hygiene routines. Then make sure to demonstrate how to properly use these tools and devices to ensure the safety and independence of your patients who need them.

Another part of this section is post-mortem care. Here, you will prepare the body of the deceased before the viewing of the family. This includes washing the body, drying the body, taking out all connected medical equipment, proper positioning of the body parts, and covering the body with a shroud. You must also place an identification tag on the toe of the deceased before the body is transported to the morgue.

Rest and Sleep

For this final section in the category, it's all about your role in promoting your patient's rest and sleep. You must evaluate the sleeping needs of your patients and intervene accordingly. To do this, apply your knowledge of your patients to promote the proper interventions for rest and sleep. You may also have to schedule patient care activities which promote sufficient rest for the patients and minimize the factors in your patients' environments which may be disturbing their rest.

Adequate rest and sleep are vital to the overall recovery and health of patients suffering from any medical disease or condition. Without enough rest and sleep, this will hurt the psychological and physical well-being of the patient. The rest and sleep needed by patients would vary depending on their activity levels, wellness levels, developmental stages, and ages. However, you must also remember that the rest and sleeping needs of patients who suffer from illnesses or diseases will increase. If during your assessment, you discover that your patient suffers from a sleep disorder, you may employ the proper interventions which will specifically address that disorder. To help you with this, you may ask your patient to keep a sleep log. Other helpful tools include a subjective sleep history, polysomnography, and a complete physical examination.

Depending on the sleep disorder of your patient, you may utilize your pathophysiology knowledge to help your patient get enough rest and sleep. For this, you may employ many interventions such as pharmacologic measures, non-pharmacological measures, and even assistive devices. You must also help your patient establish a good routine of sleep hygiene. This will help them rest better while you're taking care of them. Then provide your patients with a template to guide them when it's time for them to go home.

Chapter 3: Category Review Guide for Health Promotion and Maintenance

Looking at this category from a nursing perspective, it means that nurses deal with their patients in all the aspects of their development. From the time they're developing in-utero to death, nurses deal with patients. Therefore, your role as a nurse is to identify the norms in the patient's development, promote healthy behaviors, detect diseases early, and to intervene as needed. This category contains a lot of information which we can further divide into three main groups or topics.

The first topic to focus on is human development. Here, you need to learn about normal patterns in the development of human beings. From newborn babies to senior adults, it's important for you to know the common changes the body undergoes as it ages. This is vital so you can detect any medical conditions early and initiate interventions as soon as possible. You should be able to distinguish what's normal from what's not in terms of development. Apart from the physical development, it's also important to know about the emotional, cognitive, and social development of patients across their lifespan.

The next main topic under this category is the physical assessment. You must have a good understanding of the proper way to perform assessments of the physical systems of your patients. After your assessment, you must also know whether your findings are normal or abnormal. As a nurse, it's important for you to select the appropriate techniques for the physical assessments of your patients and translate your findings into the required nursing interventions.

The final topic to think about is self-care and optimal states of health. As a nurse, you must encourage your patients to learn self-care to promote their optimal states of health. For this topic, you need to learn more about the identification of high-risk behaviors, the important actions which are related to chronic medical conditions, the lifestyle factors which affect health, and the proper health screenings to perform on patients for the varying stages of life. Read on to learn more about this category.

The Basic Concepts Covered in Health Promotion and Maintenance

This is another important category for you to review before taking the NCLEX-RN. Here, the topics focus on the principles of growth and development, learning how to detect health problems early, preventing illnesses, and educating your patients on how they can achieve optimal health. This category accounts for about 9% of the NCLEX-RN questions.

The Aging Process

The process of aging starts from when we are born, and it slowly progresses to when we reach our senior years. As a nurse, it's important to understand the various aging stages so that you can apply your knowledge to care for and educate your patients appropriately. For each stage of development, the aging process differs. Each of these stages has its developmental milestones, warning signs which may indicate abnormalities, and special needs you must consider when you're planning for the care of your patients and communicating with them. Here are the different stages:

- **Infancy:** from birth - 12 months

- **Preadolescence:** 2 stages

    o **Preschool:** 1 year - 4 years

    o **School-age:** 5 years - 12 years

- **Adolescence:** 13 years - 18 years (this is where puberty starts)

- **Adulthood:** 3 stages

    o **Working years:** 19 years - 64 years

    o **Retirement years:** 65 years - 85 years

    o **Senior years / Elderly:** 86 years and above

Birth Process

Nowadays, it's important to monitor pregnancies from when the mother first learns that she is with the child until a couple of weeks after the child is born. This ensures that you will be able to provide the best possible health outcomes for both the infant and the mother. Let's discuss the topics under this section:

- **Antepartum care**

This may also be referred to as prenatal care. It involves you collecting relevant information about the mother's medical history, her current health state, her health information, and any counseling which may affect the outcome of the mother's pregnancy. This type of care occurs before the child is born.

- **Calculation of delivery date**

One of the first questions asked by expecting women is the due date of her baby. You can calculate the estimated due date of delivery via Naegele's Rule. Base the calculation on the first day of the mother's last menstrual period. Of course, this calculation only gives an estimate of the baby's due date. Only 4% of infants are born on this estimated date. A pregnancy is considered full term if the baby was born between 37 – 42 weeks. If the baby is born before this, he/she is considered premature. And if the pregnancy lasts for more than 42 weeks, this is considered overdue.

- **Cultural considerations**

You must also find out the cultural and religious practices and backgrounds of your patients. This is because varying cultures have different views and beliefs about pregnancy and the process of giving birth. Make yourself familiar with these customs, accept them, and accommodate your patients the best way you can.

- **Danger signs**

You must also look for the danger signs which may indicate life-threatening or severe conditions for both the mother and the baby. Make sure to watch out for signs such as:

- a decrease in fetal movement after the 24th week of pregnancy;

- constant headaches, especially during the last trimester;

- dimmed or blurred vision during

the last trimester;

- severe swelling or a sudden onset of swelling of the feet and hands, especially during the last trimester;

- severe abdominal pain that's unrelenting; or

- vaginal bleeding.

- **The health of the fetus**

It's also important for you to provide the mothers with the relevant information they need for them to monitor the health of their babies. For instance, they must feel the first fetal movements around the 17th to the 19th week of their pregnancy. These movements may provide information regarding the health of the fetus, especially during the later pregnancy stages. It's also important to take note of the heart rate of the fetus every time the mother comes in for a prenatal visit.

- **The health of the mother**

An important aspect of prenatal care is to document the past health history and the current state of health of the mother. This documentation must include information regarding the mother's medications, blood pressure, genetic history, weight, family, and lifestyle. In particular, all of the medications must be listed and carefully administered. Otherwise, instead of helping, the medications might cause a miscarriage or hurt the fetus' development.

- **Nutrition of mother and baby**

It's important for you to provide nutritional counseling as a part of the mother's prenatal care. This helps ensure that the mother acquires all of the proper nutrients she needs to ensure the healthy development of the baby. This may also help reduce the risk of postpartum and intrapartum morbidity. In the case of pregnant teenagers, they need more calcium, phosphorus, and protein since their bodies are still in the process of growth and development too.

- **Rh factor**

Testing for the Rh factor is another important aspect of prenatal care. You won't need to perform any intervention if both parents lack the Rh factor or if only the mother has the Rh factor. But if the mother lacks the Rh factor while the father has this factor or if the Rh status of the father isn't known, then you may have to administer a dose of RhoGAM (Rho immune globulin) to the mother in her 28th week. This helps prevent any immune-mediated complications at birth or in the later stages of the pregnancy.

- **Routine tests**

Throughout the prenatal period, several routine tests may be done on the mother. One of the most important types of non-invasive tests is ultrasound. This confirms the viability of the fetus, the gestational age, and the placenta's location. You can also use this test to monitor the growth and anatomy of the fetus. On the other hand, an important type of invasive test is amniocentesis. This test can provide you with detailed information regarding any chromosomal or genetic abnormalities of the developing fetus.

Intrapartum Care

This type of care refers to what you would give to a mother from the time she starts with her labor up to the time when the infant is born. There are three major factors which trigger a pregnant woman's labor which is the effect of oxytocin, the distension of her uterus, and the effect of her hormones. The most common signs that labor is about to begin are when the woman's amniotic membranes rupture and when she loses her cervical mucus plug. Once labor starts, you must be able to identify the different labor stages to provide the proper interventions needed for each of these stages:

- **4 cm – 10 cm dilation**

During this stage, the woman's cervix continues to efface and dilate. The interventions to perform here are monitoring, documenting the process, and evaluating the need for analgesia.

- **Full dilation to delivery**

As the infant goes down to the birth canal, your evaluation must include any changes in the woman's perineum which are an indication that the birth is about to happen. Such changes include crowning, visibility of the baby's body parts, bulging or an increase in the bloody show. You must also monitor the mother and baby's vital signs along with how the baby's head is positioned in the birth canal.

- **Delivery of the baby to the delivery of the placenta**

Usually, the placenta gets delivered between

5-to minutes after the birth of the baby. You must check the umbilical cord for one vein and two arteries.

- **Recovery**

It's important to frequently check the mother's uterus for the tone and position, especially for the first 60 minutes after giving birth. Around 2 hours after giving birth, you must evaluate the mother's fundal height, vital signs, and any vaginal discharge or bleeding. You must also check the mother's bladder for any distention. If needed, you may also have to help with breastfeeding, especially for new mothers.

Postpartum Care

After the mother gives birth to the baby, you need to continuously monitor her for any signs of complications such as:

- **Hemorrhage**

Explain to the mother that it's completely normal for her to experience some bleeding mixed with her vaginal discharge for about 3-6 weeks after her delivery. Evaluate the patient for any abnormal bleeding and educate her as well so she can evaluate herself when she gets home. It's important to look for intense spurts of bleeding or passing large clots.

- **Illness and infection**

It's also important to monitor the temperatures of mothers who have just given birth. An increase in temperature may indicate an infection. Other signs of infection to watch out for are cough; chest pain; smelly or copious vaginal discharge; perineal pain; red, tender or warm breasts; painful urination or pain that may or may not be accompanied by swelling.

Neonatal Care

This type of care is given to newborn infants. Right after the baby comes out of the mother, you must evaluate his/her vital signs, breathing, and overall appearance. This will help you determine if you need to perform any interventions. After this initial evaluation, check for:

- **APGAR Score**

This refers to an overall number which you can determine from the individual scores you've taken from the assessments you performed a minute after the infant's birth. These assessments include the color/appearance, the pulse/heart rate, the reflex irritability/grimace, the muscle tone/activity, and the respiratory effort/respiration. In each of these assessments, you would give a score from 0-2. The higher the score is, the better.

- **Newborn care**

This is especially important for first-time mothers. You must educate them on how to care for their newborn babies. You may have to answer the mother's questions about basic care, feeding, bathing, caring for the umbilical cord, and building the parent-child bond. You may also have to discuss the basic safety concerns such as sleep positioning, visitors, car seats, and more.

- **Warning signs of complications**

You must also monitor the infants while they're in the nursery and while they're with their new mothers to see if there are any signs which indicate complications of health issues after birth. Some of these warning signs include bulging or sunken-in cranial soft spots; a high fever; vomiting more than once within 24 hours; the inability to keep down water and food or breathing difficulties.

In some cases, you may also have to provide counseling to the new mothers with regards to contraception since their menstrual cycles may come back within 6-8 weeks after giving birth. For mothers who are breastfeeding, this period may be a bit longer. Some mothers may also experience a postpartum period which can be extremely stressful. Therefore, you must inform and educate them on the possible interventions if they notice frequent emotional swings after the 2nd or 3rd postpartum week.

Developmental Transitions and Stages

In each of the developmental phases, there are standard expectations for emotional, cognitive, social, and physical growth that you need to be aware of. You must know the developmental milestones of each stage, their needs, and any warning signs which may indicate abnormal growth and development.

- **Infants**

Physically speaking, infants must be able to suckle well and grasp an object as a reflex when placed in their palms. They should also be able to focus on an object for a short time. Most infants may have swollen genitalia or breasts, milia on their faces, and heads which are slightly misshapen but which become more round as they age. As they grow older, infants must learn how to grasp with their index finger and thumb, vocalize, and respond selectively to words spoken to them.

It's important for infants to be able to form bonds with their caregivers and, of course, their parents. The warning signs to look out for in infants include not being able to transfer objects from one hand to another by the time they reach nine months or not being able to roll from their tummy to their side by the time they reach ten months.

- **Preschool**

Children in this age group must be able to enjoy physical activities. Their physical coordination must be greater, and they should start exhibiting fine motor skills. Preschool children should be able to undress and dress themselves; manipulate and utilize small objects using their fingers and hands, and exhibit progressive control over their bladders and bowel movements.

Also, preschool children are already aware of limits. They may frequently say "no" and must have a vocabulary between 500-3,000 words.

They should be able to speak in short sentences, use a pencil to draw the basic shapes, and are always eager to please the people closest to them.

In terms of needs, preschool children need a lot of consistency and routine. They should feel secure in their environments. At the same time, they require close supervision, especially in harmful environments. Parents must also allow children in this age group to exert their independence and have unstructured playtime.

For this age group, look out for abnormal or delayed developmental signs such as not being able to walk by the time the child reaches 18 months; not being able to say a minimum of 15 words; not being able to imitate actions or words; not being able to follow simple instructions; not wanting to play with other children; not taking part in "pretend play;" and focusing too much on mature subject matter such as violence.

- **School-age**

For children in this age group, they have a more advanced level of physical coordination which means that they should already be able to perform various activities with a combination of movements. They should also be able to follow more complex commands with more than just one step. School-age children must be able to retain more information and remember more details about themselves such as their full name, age, and even their address.

In terms of needs, you may have to perform an early intervention for school-age children who have hearing or vision problems. Such issues manifest as soon as they start school. Also, conditions such as a lateral curvature of the spine or scoliosis may start developing at this age. It's important to catch this condition early to provide the appropriate intervention.

For children in this age group, look out for warning signs such as continued bed wetting or being unable to express or verbalize the anxiety they feel at home or in school.

- **Adolescence**

Children in this age group are commonly struggling to find their sense of identity. They tend to form strong bonds with their peers, and it's normal for them to perform risky behaviors. Physically speaking, they undergo several changes such as the development of their secondary sexual characteristics, an increase in their hormone production, along with a concern with and a growing interest in physical attractiveness.

Because of the many physical changes experienced by the children in this age group, they may feel distressed or overwhelmed. Therefore, you need to prepare them for these changes and talk to them about what they are to expect at this time. In some cases, adolescents may even experience changes in their personality and mood swings because of these changes. When looking for warning signs, take note of persistent misbehavior or excessive aggressiveness, especially when these behaviors are displayed at the school.

- **Working adults**

People in this age group are trying to find the purpose or meaning in their lives through their relationships, families, and work. According to the Psychosocial Development Theory of Erikson states that this stage is to "resolve the conflict of intimacy versus isolation." Working adults either focus on finding the right partner and starting their own family or deciding to remain single. According to the same theory, at the age of 35 up until adults turn 64, they work to "resolve the conflict of generativity versus stagnation." Adults can find more meaning in the career they've chosen, and they're looking for ways to leave a lasting legacy behind.

In terms of their physique, adults in this age group are considered to be in the "prime of their lives" from 25-25 years of age. After that, some adults might start developing chronic medical conditions. In such cases, you need to intervene and suggest the appropriate lifestyle modifications to treat or manage these conditions.

The needs of the adults in this age group can either negatively or positively influence their functioning and development. When looking for warning signs, check for those adults who have substance abuse issues or those who feel that their life is meaningless.

- **Retired adults**

The adults in this age group begin to experience a gradual decline in terms of their physical functioning. Most of them will retire from their work. In some cases, retired adults may even experience a gradual decline in their cognitive functioning too. According to Erikson's Theory, the adults in this age group need to "resolve the conflict of ego integrity or despair." When retired adults look back on their lives, they either feel despair or a sense of accomplishment.

Also, the adults in this group may start experiencing changes in terms of their interpersonal relationships. This may be because of a decline in their functions, illnesses, and seeing the people they know, die. It can be very challenging for retired adults to transition to life without work. They may also experience hardships due to the loss of or changes in their close personal relationships. For the warning signs, look for those who feel regret or despair about their lives instead of feeling a sense of peace or pride with how they lived their lives.

- **Elderly**

People in this age group are likely to show a progressive decline both in their cognitive and physical functioning. Also, they will likely experience a significant loss in terms of their interpersonal relationships. The elderly must always learn to find meaning and acceptance in their lives. Otherwise, you might see the warning signs such as having suicidal behaviors or thoughts in the elderly.

Health Promotion and Disease Prevention

By definition, health is the absence of illness

and disease. But in reality, there are a lot of people who enjoy a healthy life even though they're dealing with health challenges. So perhaps, it's more appropriate to use the term "health and wellness" when representing a state of emotional, social and physical well-being. Nurses play an important role in empowering and educating patients so that they can take control of their health. As a nurse, you can help your patients find all of the health resources needed based on their disabilities or specific medical conditions. Therefore, you must be aware of the programs which are part of health promotion and disease prevention:

- **Cessation of smoking**

There are many reasons why people keep on smoking even though they know all of the bad effects of this habit. And once a person starts this habit, it can be very difficult for them to quit. To promote the successful cessation of smoking, you may have to employ more than just one strategy for your patients.

- **Exercise**

This is another important aspect of the health and wellness of your patients. No matter what age groups your patients are in or what activity level they have, exercising is essential. Exercise can improve the functions of the respiratory and cardiovascular functions, assist in the maintenance of a healthy weight, stimulate the metabolism, improve the quality of sleep, strengthen the bones, and enhance the overall flexibility, balance, endurance, and strength of your patients.

- **The health of the breasts**

It's important to educate your female patients on how to perform a breast self-examination as soon as they reach puberty. They must do this at least once a month to stay safe.

- **The health of the testicles**

One of the most curable types of solid tumors is testicular cancer, and this is very common in men aged 15 – 35. It's important to educate your male patients on how to perform a testicular self-examination. If they happen to find any abnormalities in their testicles, they must consult with their doctor right away.

- **Hormone Replacement Therapy or HRT**

Women who are either perimenopausal or menopausal are potential candidates for this type of therapy. This is important to help manage any negative symptoms of these conditions such as vaginal dryness, sweating, and hot flashes. However, before recommending HRT, discuss all of the benefits as well as the risks with your patients.

- **Immunizations**

Immunizations are an important aspect of health throughout the lifetime of patients. Most immunizations are given when people are either in the preschool or school-age. However, there are also some types of immunizations which are given to adults such as pneumococcal pneumonia, meningococcal, and more.

- **Mental health**

Often, nurses are the ones who deal with patients more intimately compared to other members of the healthcare team. In some cases, you might be the first one to notice any mental health issues in patients or those who may be at risk for developing anxiety, depression, and more. In such cases, you may provide your patients with tips on how to manage their stress effectively. You may also help them arrange care, especially for those who need intervention to maintain their mental health.

- **Nutrition**

Nutrition is crucial for the health and wellness of your patients. Although sensible eating is always recommended, keep in mind that some of your patients may need to follow special types of diets. For instance, patients suffering from hypertension must avoid eating foods which are high in sodium such as processed or canned foods. Also, patients who have osteoporosis must consume more foods which are high in calcium. And those who have diabetes need to restrict their carbohydrate intake, and more. Therefore, you must make yourself aware of the conditions of your patients to recommend the proper diet and nutrition for them.

- **Oral health**

It's important to emphasize the importance of oral health as it is linked to other physical diseases. For one, periodontal disease or gum disease is linked to heart disease, diabetes, and other types of chronic, inflammatory conditions.

- **Other types of therapies**

In some cases, your patients may want to incorporate other types of therapies along with western medicine. Such therapies include hypnosis, massage, acupuncture, and more. Some patients may also take their supplements, homeopathic therapies, essential oils, and more to enhance the effects of their treatments. Also, some patients may even seek consultation from other types of medical practitioners such as chiropractors and shamans.

- **Prevention of stroke and heart disease**

As a nurse, it's your responsibility to identify any abnormalities in your patient's blood pressure since high blood pressure is commonly associated with stroke and heart disease. For those who have a high risk, you may encourage them to monitor their blood pressure even at home. You can also make your patients aware of the symptoms as well as the normal parameters for diastolic and systolic blood pressures.

- **Skin health**

It's essential to speak to your patients about the harmful effects of excessive UV exposure as well as the importance of having regular screenings for skin cancer. You may also provide your patients with helpful tips to maintain skin health such as wearing protective clothing, using sunscreen, and more.

- **Weight management**

When promoting the healthy management of weight, concentrate on the incremental modifications which help move your patients towards a healthy weight for their build and height. Even a modest amount of weight loss can have a significant impact on your patients, especially those who suffer from chronic illnesses.

Health Screening

Knowing all about health screening allows you to serve your patients better. This topic requires you to have a combined knowledge of pathophysiology along with the known risk factors for certain age or ethnic groups. The main health screening tests you would have to learn about or perform include:

- **Blood Sugar**

You can check the blood sugar levels of fasting or non-fasting patient. If your patient has been fasting for over 8 hours and you get a level higher than 125 mg/dL, you may need to perform further tests. On the other hand, a patient who hasn't been fasting must have a level below 199 mg/dL.

- **Blood Pressure**

By definition, normal blood pressure is any value below 120/80 mm Hg. There are many subcategories of hypertension namely stage I, stage UU, and elevated. There is also a condition known as severe hypertension which is defined as a value above 140/90 mm Hg. Hypertension is known as a "silent killer" because it can be asymptomatic even when severe. The other risk factors for high blood pressure include hyperlipidemia, an inactive lifestyle, and an age above 60.

- **Colorectal Screening**

Adults aged 50 and above must have this screening done regularly. This includes numerous tests namely a digital rectal exam, sigmoidoscopy, double-contrast barium enema, fecal occult blood testing, digital rectal exam, and colonoscopy. For those who have a history of colorectal cancer, they must have screenings more frequently and at an earlier age.

- **Fasting Lipid Profile**

Adults must have this test done every five

years. Normal values include a total cholesterol level below 200 mg/dL, fatty acid or triglyceride level below 150 mg/dL, low-density lipoprotein level below 100 mg/dL, and high-density lipoprotein level above 50 mg/dL in women and 40 mg/dL in men.

- **Mammogram**

Women who are between the age of 40-50 years old must have a baseline mammogram done. Then yearly screenings are recommended for most women until they reach the age of 55. These tests can be done either annually or biannually. But if the woman has a family history of breast cancer, it's recommended to have this done earlier.

- **Prostate Screening**

Men at the age of 50 and above must have this screening done regularly. There is a specific blood test which measures the prostate-specific antigen of the men. Another test that is used for this screening is the digital rectal exam.

High-Risk Behavior

Another important aspect of Health Promotion and Maintenance is to document the history of your patients, especially those who are likely to engage in lifestyles or behaviors which have a high risk and which might increase their risk of developing certain illnesses, injuries, diseases or even death. A lot of patients aren't even aware that they're at risk so you must educate them as part of your comprehensive healthcare plan. Some of the most common high-risk behaviors include:

- **Accident-related**

For a lot of the age groups, the number one cause of death is unintended injuries. For this, you may provide counseling on how your patients may reduce this risk by using seatbelts while in moving vehicles, using protective gear such as helmets, and more.

- **Sexually-related**

Unprotected vaginal, oral or anal sexual activities may increase a patient's risk of getting STDs or HIV/AIDs. These might also result in unplanned pregnancies. Therefore, you have to educate your patients on how to use barrier protection or contraception methods, especially for those who plan to have several sexual partners.

Lifestyle Choices

The lifestyle choices of patients vary. They have their own set of characteristics or actions which may range from intentional decisions to routine habits. Each of these decisions and habits may affect the health of your patient either positively or negatively depending on their current health circumstances.

Your patients may also have their self-care activities which they perform to either enhance or promote their well-being and health. These are known as "self-care" practices because they are done without the supervision of medical professionals. But for elderly patients or those who either have physical or developmental disabilities, they may need your assistance to perform these activities adequately.

Physical Assessment Techniques

The "History of Present Illness" and "Health Histories" of patients are the subjective descriptions of your patient's health circumstances and symptoms. On the other hand, a physical assessment provides you with objective information about your patient's physical condition. Both these descriptions will be very helpful in your decision-making, especially in terms of determining the proper intervention. Here are the basic physical assessment techniques to use when assessing patients:

- **Auscultation**

This method involves the use of a stethoscope to listen to fluid and air movements inside your patient's body. Use the bell of the stethoscope to listen to low-frequency sounds. Use the diaphragm of the stethoscope to listen to high-frequency sounds.

- **Inspection**

This is also known as purposeful observation, and it contains a lot of important information about the general health of your patient. Inspection involves your patient's movements, posture, speech, and body habitus. All of these can tell you more about your patient's personal care habits, nutritional status, and can even provide you with indications about abnormalities in terms of your patient's development. Checking your patient's vital signs is also an important aspect of inspection. Sometimes, you may have to customize the assessment technique depending on your patient.

• Palpation

This is when you use both of your fingertips and your palms to apply light, moderate or deep pressure to specific internal structures. The purpose of this assessment technique is to collect information about your patient's state and function. Through this technique, you can assess the quality, rhythm, and rate of your patient's pulse. You can also use palpation to detect a cardiac thrill or even displaced, swollen or tender internal organs or bones. Finally, this assessment can also provide you with information about the fluid status or hydration of your patient by checking for signs of edema or skin turgor.

• Percussion

This technique provides you with information about your patient's levels of fluid and air within his/her body cavity or organs. To do this, press your middle finger over a specific structure while using the middle and index finger of your other hand to tap lightly on your pressed middle finger. The sound that comes back to you can either be loud/hollow if air is present or soft/dull is exudate or fluid is present. This technique is often used to assess conditions involving the abdomen or chest cavity.

Chapter 4: Category Review Guide for Management of Care

We've already gone through how the most important goal of the NCLEX-RN is to determine whether or not you're ready to start performing as an entry-level nurse. When you're already a nurse, and you're on your shift, it's quite common to have to manage patients with several, complicated care plans. Therefore, you must be able to determine which aspects of patient care are most important to ensure positive and safe patient outcomes. It's also important for you to understand your responsibilities and legal rights in different types of care environments to protect yourself and your patients.

For this category, most of the NCLEX-RN questions are focused on the needs of patients. These are meant to evaluate your knowledge of the different topics included in this category along with your ability to analyze and to apply your knowledge to different types of situations.

Of course, there are also some questions which aren't directly related to patient care. You may also have to answer questions about what you must do if you see any unsafe behaviors and practices in the workplace. Such questions will show how well you understand the whole scope of ethical and legal responsibilities in the nursing practice.

Basic Concepts Covered in Management of Care

This category makes up most of the questions on the test as it contains about 20% of the total items in the NCLEX-RN. This percentage shows how relevant the topic is. It focuses on directing and providing nursing care while protecting yourself, your patients, and the other members of the healthcare team.

Advance Directives

Advance directives refer to a legal document which contains the wishes of your patients with regards to their care in cases where they aren't able to communicate independently. Some examples of these directives are healthcare proxies, organ donation plans, living wills, and others. Let's take a look at more detailed examples of advance directives:

- **Self-Determination**

Back in the year 1990, Congress has passed the "Patient Self-Determination Act." In this bill, health institutions such as hospitals, home health agencies, nursing homes, and others, must advise their patients of their right to either refuse or accept care. These patients must also be advised on their advance directive options. If your patient already created an advance directive, you may help by documenting this fact in his chart. If not, you may have to educate your patients on what these are and talk about your patient's future healthcare goals.

- **Life Planning**

One of the main purposes of having advance directives is to ensure that you or other members of the healthcare team will carry out all of the wishes of the patient. It's your responsibility to incorporate your patient's advance directives into the healthcare plan. You must also ask for a copy of your patient's advance directives so you can attach it to your patient's chart.

Advocacy

Your advocacy is at the very heart of your nursing profession. This refers to promoting the interests of your patients or acting on behalf of them. Nurses are advocates for patients. You have diverse duties which may include having to explain medical procedures to your patients and the members of their family; making sure that your patient's care plan is safely executed and in a timely manner; and serving as a comprehensive source of information and a means of communication between the other members of the healthcare team. In some cases, you may have to ask for advice or seek the opinions of the other people involved in the care of your patients, such as his/her dietician or social worker.

Assignment, Delegation, and Supervision

These are essential skills any nurse must have. No matter how efficient or amazing you are, there will always be times when you need to ask for help in order to accomplish all of the required tasks for the care of your patient every day. To be able to delegate tasks successfully, you must find the right person to delegate the tasks to. Then, it's your job to explain the task clearly. Finally, it's also your responsibility to provide supervision and support to get the best possible outcome.

When it comes to delegation, there are certain tasks which you should never assign to non-professionals. Such tasks include nursing examinations and assessments; diagnosis of conditions; progress plans or care goals; or interventions which require advanced skills, training or knowledge. Before you begin delegating or assigning tasks, think about these five questions:

- Is it proper for this task to be delegated?

- Is the person you're planning to delegate the task to qualified?

- Is your patient stable enough and can you predict the outcome of the task you're planning to delegate?

- Have you explained the task clearly and have you given the proper instructions?

- Will you be able to supervise the task

until it's an accomplishment?

The most acceptable types of tasks to delegate to other people are those who are "routine" or which don't have changing protocols. Some examples are dressing, bathing, feeding, transferring, and more. Also, you must only delegate tasks for stable patients. It's never a good idea to delegate tasks involving unpredictable or unstable patients. Neither is it a good idea to delegate tasks which require complex knowledge or complex skills.

In the workplace, nurses are also considered as leaders. This means that you must learn how to unite your team so everyone works together to reach one goal and that is to provide the best care to all of your patients.

Apart from delegation and assignment, you may also have to supervise different types of nursing staff such as licensed vocational nurses, other registered nurses, nursing active personnel, and licensed practical nurses. You might even have the responsibility of coordinating the tasks of your entire nursing team. To supervise efficiently, you must be able to coordinate clearly, follow-up regularly, listen actively, have good problem-solving and conflict-resolution skills, and have adequate technical knowledge of everything you're supervising. You may also have to evaluate the abilities and skills of those you've supervised and provided constructive criticism if necessary.

Case Management

As a nurse, you're also responsible for the development, implementation, and revision of your the care plans of your patients. You must make sure that these plans will help your patients reach their health goals and be able to maintain their health even after they've been discharged independently.

Case management doesn't just involve the care of your patient while in your medical facility. Part of this is helping your patients find and make use of all the available post-care resources. It's your job to help your patients achieve this by identifying their individual needs and talking to them about their health goals. Successful case management ensures the safety of the patients and considers all of the cost-effective options for them too.

Whenever possible, you must also incorporate any findings based on evidence into the care plans of your patients. To do this, you must keep yourself updated with the current studies and research. This will help you stay up-to-date so that you can give helpful recommendations to your patients. Also, you may want to consult with other professionals whom you know may help you with your case management.

Care plans of patients tend to evolve depending on how they respond to the interventions you're performing. Therefore, it's also your responsibility to make revisions to their care plans as needed. Communicate regularly with your patients whenever you're making any changes to avoid any misunderstandings.

Patient Rights

Apart from educating your patients and explaining things to them, it's also your responsibility to inform them of their rights as patients when they are admitted to your healthcare facility. Here are some of the most important patient rights to discuss with your patients:

- **HIPAA**

The Health Insurance Portability and Accountability Act or HIPAA is meant to protect the personal and medical information of your patients. Therefore, only those who are directly involved in their medical care, case management or insurance reimbursement may have access to this information.

- **Patient's Bill of Rights**

This is a document which specifies the rights and responsibilities of each patient as recipients of healthcare:

- **Access to Emergency Services** refers to the right to obtain evaluation as well as stabilization from emergency services wherever and whenever needed. Such services must be provided even without authorization and without financial penalty.

- **Choice of Plans and Providers** refers to the right of the patient to select healthcare providers who give high-quality care as needed

- **Complaints and Appeals** refer to the right a fair, objective, and fast review of any complaints against a patient's healthcare provider, healthcare plan, healthcare facility or healthcare personnel.

- **Confidentiality of Health Information** refers to the right of the patient to speak with healthcare providers in private and keep all of his healthcare information private too.

- **Consumer Responsibilities** specify that patients must share all relevant information about their past illnesses and medications to their healthcare providers.

- **Information Disclosure** refers to the right to easily and accurately understand information about the patient's health plans, the healthcare facilities, and the healthcare providers.

- **Participation in Treatment Decisions** refers to the right of the patient to be informed of all possible treatment options so that they can make decisions about their care. This right also applied to the other healthcare proxies of the patient if he isn't able to decide for himself.

As a nurse, it's your responsibility to make sure that your patients understand all of these rights and responsibilities. You also have to evaluate the knowledge and understanding of the other members of the healthcare team in case the patient wants to ask them questions about these rights and responsibilities.

Collaboration

In terms of Management of Care, collaboration refers to the interdisciplinary action between the different aspects of healthcare. As a nurse, you will be working with social workers, physicians, pharmacists, dieticians, and several other healthcare professionals to give your patient the best possible care. Collaboration involves teamwork, cohesiveness, and integration.

In most cases, you will have the most intimate contact with patients. Therefore, you must prepare yourself to start these interdisciplinary communications based on the information given by your patients and your observations. In other words, you act as the central contact point of the whole collaborative healthcare team.

Management

Often, you would also be acting as the manager of your patient's healthcare team. Therefore, you must be aware of all the roles, duties, and responsibilities of each of the team members. You will act as the liaison between your patient and his healthcare team. You're the first person who will encounter problems, so you need to know how to solve them. You may also have to use conflict-resolution skills to settle any issues between your patient, the team, and the individual members of the team. It would be helpful for you to create an overall strategy which you will use whenever you need to handle problems.

Confidentiality and Information Security

Your role as a nurse also includes maintaining the confidentiality of your patients and taking the necessary steps to ensure that their privacy is always maintained. To do this effectively, you must have a comprehensive understanding of the HIPAA. Make sure that only those who are authorized have access to the personal, medical, and sensitive information of your patients. If you discover any breach from other members of your healthcare team, you must take the necessary intervention right away.

Continuity of Care

This refers to the proper and adequate communication of relevant information between the various agencies and departments. This ensures that everybody involved with the patient understands and agrees with the healthcare goals of that patient. You must have a good knowledge of the proper procedures and guidelines for admitting, transferring, and discharging patients to and from your healthcare facility.

You must also be familiar with all of the required forms and referral paperwork which are part of your patient's medical record. If your patient has any unresolved health issues, it's also your responsibility to follow-up or forward all of the information to the different departments or agencies which need it. At times, you might also have to prepare reports for the reference of the patient's new healthcare team.

Priorities

Each day, nurses must learn how to prioritize. You need to establish the healthcare priorities of all your patients individually and all your patients collectively. There are plenty of guidelines and frameworks to use when you're trying to develop or establish priorities. These include:

- **ABCs** which refer to the airway, breathing, and circulatory or cardiovascular system.

- **Agency Policies** which refer to the protocols dictated by your healthcare facility regulations.

- **Maslow's Hierarchy** which refers to the patient's physiologic needs, then his security and safety, then his sense of belonging and love, then his self-actualization and self-esteem.

- **Medication Indicators** which refer to

managing your patient's care according to the medications your patients need to take and when they need to take those medications.

- **Patient Activity** which refers to your reports which, in turn, are essential tools when you're planning your daily priorities. Also, you may have to make modifications in your priorities depending on the activities and needs of your patients. This will help you accomplish all that you need to do efficiently.

- **Patient and Family** which refers to you taking some time to understand all of your patients and their family members. This will help you in your assessment of your patient's needs and be able to prioritize your daily care duties well.

- **Time** which refers to your efficiency in time management and being able to delegate tasks as needed.

Your ability to assess your patients and prioritize their needs based on these assessments will allow you to think of the required interventions. These will also allow you to provide care to your patients who require immediate attention or those who remain unstable. This is especially important if you have several patients under your care. When thinking about priorities, those who have the following conditions must be at the top of your list:

- Post-surgery patients need to be monitored regularly and given pain and fluid management.

- Baseline status deterioration wherein any changes from the baseline would need immediate assessment and intervention to sustain the life of the patient.

- Shock is a condition which needs targeted intervention depending on the cause. You may also have to implement specific measures to reverse any physiologic changes the shock triggered.

- Allergic reactions require immediate interventions in the form of pharmacological medications.

- Chest pain requires immediate monitoring of the patient's cardiac activity or cardiovascular deterioration, and the appropriate pharmacologic intervention.

- Post-diagnostic procedures require temporary but close and frequent monitoring.

- Other unusual symptoms require further assessment and monitoring for any changes or worsening of your patient's symptoms.

- Malfunctioning equipment also requires immediate attention, especially if these are connected to unstable patients.

Ethical Practice

Each day, you need to make use of the basic principles of ethics and morals when making judgments and when determining whether what you're doing is right or wrong. The ANA or American Nurses Association has its own Code of Ethics which you need to make yourself familiar with. The code contains all of the ethical guidelines which define the standards and values for nurses. To give you a better idea of this code, here are some of the most important ethical principles:

- **Accountability** which refers to owning up to your actions.

- **Autonomy** which refers to a patient's right to make decisions independently.

- **Beneficence** which refers to performing actions in the best interest of your patients.

- **Confidentiality** which refers to keeping your patient's personal, medical, and sensitive information private.

- **Fidelity** which refers to maintaining your faithfulness to all of the ethical principles and the Code of Ethics.

- **Justice** which refers to providing all of your patients with fair, impartial, and equal treatment.

- **Nonmaleficence** which refers to behaving in such a way that you avoid any harm.

- **Virtues** which refer to the nursing standards namely compassion, honesty, trustworthiness, and integrity.

Informed Consent

This means that you have discussed all of the benefits and risks of a specific treatment plan or procedure with your patients before they agree to it. Informed consent has four important components mainly:

- explaining the treatment or procedure to the patient in full detail;

- explaining all of the benefits of the treatment or procedure in full detail;

- discussing all of the possible alternative treatments or procedures; and

- discussing all of the potential ramifications if your patient doesn't agree to the treatment or procedure suggested.

Your job is to facilitate this process. In doing this, you may have to evaluate whether or not your patient has the capacity to give informed consent. If not (like in cases where your patient is a minor or isn't mentally competent), you need to identify the appropriate person who will act on your patient's behalf. In some cases, you may even have to be the witness to informed consent. Then you must make sure that this consent happens before the suggested procedure or treatment. Finally, you also need to make sure to document the refusal of your patient on his medical record.

Information Technology

This aspect can have a significant improvement in patient care through the quicker access of all authorized healthcare providers to all of the medical records of your patients. Information Technology can affect the safety of your patients, their health outcomes, and you can also use it for your patient's education. Consider these:

- **Electronic Health Records or EHRs**

These are computer-based charts and records of your patients. EHRs contain all of your patient's demographics, personal information, medical notes, insurance information, past medical history, immunizations, medications, vital signs, and test results. EHRs help facilitates the patient's care between authorized personnel who are part of the patient's management. This is because they permit instant access to all of the patient's required medical information. These EHRs can also indirectly or directly help with other aspects such as outcomes reporting and quality management.

- **Electronic Medication Administration Records or eMAR**

These records utilize electronic tracking systems such as barcodes to keep track of the medications of patients. Then you can use these record this information into the EHR of your patient. eMARs can improve both the safety and the outcomes of patients by significantly reducing errors in the administration of medications.

If you work with these types of IT systems in your healthcare facility, you must have a good knowledge and understanding of how they work. This is important so you will be able to use the IT systems efficiently and appropriately. One thing to remember is that when it comes to working with IT systems, the rules of patient privacy and confidentiality still apply whether you're transmitting or accessing the records of your patients.

Legal Rights and Responsibilities

As a nurse, it's also your responsibility to understand your nursing license scope of practice along with all of your legal limitations. Most of these parameters are mandated by state and federal laws and by the general guidelines such as those in the NPAs or Nurse Practice Arts. Each of the states has a Board of Nursing which serves as the credentialing body. This board also serves as the main information source regarding all the applicable laws in the state where you work.

One important aspect to remember (and try to avoid) is negligence. This refers to the failure to act or an unintentional act which ends up harming your patient. Negligence also involves your failure to act reasonably. For instance, if you aren't able to administer medication to your patient promptly and he experiences an adverse effect as a result of this failure, this is considered negligence.

Another important aspect to remember (and again, try to avoid) is malpractice. The main difference between negligence and malpractice is that the latter involves an element of intent. Often, the individual states set their requirements for malpractice which is why these requirements may vary. Generally, though, malpractice refers to when you don't competently perform all of your duties and, as a consequence, your patient gets harmed. Some examples of malpractice include giving the wrong type or the wrong dose of medication to patients.

As a nurse, it's your responsibility to provide proper care to your patients promptly. Any inappropriate or incorrect actions or even the lack of the appropriate actions may result in legal action taken against you, especially if your patient gets harmed in the process. Therefore, it's important for you to familiarize yourself with your legal responsibilities and rights:

- **Intervention During Unsafe Practices**

Apart from reporting the unsafe practices that you witness, you must also intervene if possible. That way, you can ensure the safety of your patients.

- **Patient and Staff Education**

When you participate in elective and required educational events, these will help improve your knowledge and ensure that you understand all of the ethical and legal issues.

With this comprehension, you will be able to respond appropriately as needed.

- **Patient Valuables**

Your healthcare practice or facility has its specific guidelines which you must be aware of in terms of how to handle your patient's valuables. Follow all of these guidelines to protect yourself and your patients.

- **Regulations for Reporting**

There are certain types of illnesses and health conditions such as dog bites, communicable diseases, and more which come with their own federal and state regulations which you must follow. Also, you must familiarize yourself with any regulations which apply to you like your role as a mandated reporter of crimes.

- **Response to Legal Issues**

It's your responsibility to identify any legal issues which are related to the care of your patients and respond to them appropriately.

- **Seeking Assistance**

It's your responsibility to identify any assignments and tasks which you're not qualified to perform. In such a case, it's important for you to seek guidance or assistance as needed.

- **Unsafe Practice Reporting**

If you happen to witness any unsafe practices performed by other personnel, it's your responsibility to report these both to the credentialing board of your state and to the overseeing agency.

Organ Donation

Organ donation refers to the process of taking the tissues or organs from one patient then transplanting it into or on another patient. Internal organs and other body parts such as bone marrow, bones, corneas, and even skin may be donated and transplanted. Most organ donations occur when the donor dies, but in some cases, organs are taken from living patients (such as bone marrow, kidneys, and others).

Specialized nurses are known as "procurement nurses" are the one involved in organ donation and organ transplant procedures. Even the nurses who are in charge of counseling patients and their loved ones regarding the specific details of organ donation must have had special training as required under the federal law. For entry-level nurses, you would only have to make sure that the patients aged 18 and above have a copy of their advance directives which involve organ donation in their medical records.

Quality Improvement

The different medical and healthcare institutions have their definitions of quality. Generally, though, the term "quality" refers to either meeting or exceeding the expectations of patients, the standards for care, and accomplishing all of the planned goals or outcomes for patients. Therefore, quality improvement is the process of establishing and of improving any quality issues which are related to nursing care such as:

Continuous Quality Improvement or CQI which refers to an approach to management which is focused on the assessment and improvement of any processes which have led to success.

Decision Making (Evidence-Based) which refers to an approach which is focused on making adjustments to processes and policies according to the most recent evidence from research and studies.

Nurse-Sensitive Indicators which refer to the measurements of the care of your patients which are directly affected by your nursing interventions.

Quality Management Plan and Benchmarks which refers to an approach which makes use of performance measures when making adjustments to processes and policies. The benchmarks are the points of comparison used to identify any issues in the processes and policies.

Reporting Issues where, as a nurse, you play a very important role in the improvement of quality. When you make reports about patient care issues to the right people, this ensures the proper evaluation of management which is the main reason why corrections happen.

Resources where, as a nurse, you may also be a valuable resource for your healthcare institution's quality improvement. They may use your knowledge as a data source or ask you to be part of a team that's involved in the quality improvement process. In some cases, you may also have to assess the effect of changes in processes or procedures to your nursing practices.

Total Quality Management or TQM which refers to a long-term approach to management which is focused on the satisfaction of patients.

Referrals

When taking care of your patients, you play an important role in coordinating their care with the other members of their healthcare teams or the other community agencies. Your role may be as simple as recommending a specific health provider such as a physical therapist or a dietician. Your job is to evaluate the needs of your patients correctly. After doing this, you have to assist them throughout the process of referral until they get the required care. Part of your job is to also provide all of the relevant information and documentation to the healthcare facility or provider you referred your patients to.

Chapter 5: Category Review Guide for Pharmacological and Parenteral Therapies

This category mainly involves the administration of your patients' medications, the rights of patients in terms of medication administration, and any adverse side effects of those medications. As a nurse, you must familiarize yourself with the specific situations where certain procedures and medications might hurt your patients. These are called contraindications, and they are important. When dealing with situations which involve "relative contraindication," you must approach with caution, especially when it comes to combining specific procedures and medications. It's important to remember that there are some types of medications which may improve others by increasing their potency while there are other types of medications which might negate the effects of those being taken by your patients.

Giving medications to your patients isn't the only way to treat them or improve their symptoms. For instance, patients who suffer from anemia and are starting to feel a shortness of breath won't benefit from medications. Rather, you must give such patients a blood transfusion to correct their condition. In such a case, the patient may have low hemoglobin levels which is why he/she is experiencing those symptoms. Therefore, blood transfusion is the better option. This is why you need to learn all that you can about medications and how to properly administer them to your patients.

Basic Concepts Covered in Pharmacological and Parenteral Therapies

One of your responsibilities in your nursing practice is to administer parenteral and pharmacological therapies to your patients. You must provide appropriate care to your patients in terms of administering these therapies. In the NCLEX-RN, this category accounts for 15% of the total questions.

Medication Effects

Medications are very important as have the potential to heal patients when given appropriately. Therefore, administering medications to your patients is more than simply "giving" them the pharmaceuticals. To administer properly, you need to have a broad knowledge of the different types of medications as well as their potential effects and unintended side effects. You must also know how medications interact with other drugs and therapies. A comprehensive understanding of your patient's health status is vital too so you know which medications can be tolerated and which ones can't. Let's take a look at the most important concepts in terms of medication effects:

- **Adverse or negative effects**

It's your role to monitor your patients closely and look out for any adverse or negative effects of the medication/s you've just administered. This means that you must also know what potential side effects to look out for including the physical symptoms your patients might start manifesting.

One of the most important things to be aware of are the physical signs of anaphylaxis or an allergic reaction. Apart from this, you must also need to know the steps to take when faced with life-threatening situations involving such reactions.

- **Contraindications**

Each type of medication has its list of diseases, illnesses, and conditions wherein its use is neither safe nor acceptable. It's important for you to understand all of these lists for each of the medications you are to administer to your patients. Then, as you're assessing the health status of your patient, it's time for you to correlate all of the information you have to ensure your patient's safety.

- **Interactions**

It's important to go through the complete medication history of your patient to perform a full assessment to avoid any medication interactions. This includes prescription medications, over-the-counter medications (OTCs), and herbal or natural medications as well. Remember that the prescribed fluids given to patients in hospitals have the potential to interact with their medications as well. Therefore, if any of these interactions happen, you must know the proper interventions to perform.

- **Side Effects**

Each time you administer medications to a patient, especially for the first time, you must monitor that patient for any potential or actual side effects he/she might experience. To help the process along, involve your patient in your monitoring by discussing the most common side effects to expect even before you administer the medication.

Also, familiarize yourself with all of the required countermeasures which will reduce the side effects. Finally, it's also important for you to know when it's time to consult with your patient's ordering practitioner if you think the medications need to be discontinued.

When it comes to medication administration, your role as a nurse is more than just finding out about the effects of medications and how to deal with them. You must also speak with your patients about the names of the medications, the doses you're giving, and the rationale for those medications. If your patient is taking the medications home, provide all of the proper instructions such as when your patient must take the medication and how those medications may interact with the supplements, natural remedies or other medications your patient is taking.

For outpatients, talk about the right time for them to call emergency services or when they must report any adverse reactions they're experiencing. For inpatients, it's your responsibility to decide when to consult with the ordering providers in case you see them experiencing any adverse reactions from the medications taken. Finally, it's also important for you to record all of your conversations with your patients along with your observations of how your patients react to the administered medications. Also, document the interventions you performed to either reduce or eliminate the side effects of the said medications.

Blood and Blood Products

In healthcare facilities such as hospitals, administering blood products as well as blood is a common practice. Patients may need these for different reasons such as if they're suffering from clotting deficiencies. Because of this, you require a vast knowledge of the different blood types as well as the proper administration of blood and blood products.

Before administering these fluids, the first thing you must do is properly identify your patients. There are specific guidelines which are set by the individual facilities which help reduce the errors in patient identification. Generally, though, you must take these important steps:

- Identify the correct patient then reconcile his name with the one written on the blood or blood product order.

- Check your patient's blood time and reconcile this with the blood type of the blood or blood product.

- Make sure that what you're about to infuse isn't expired.

- Finally, make sure that there is documentation for patient consent.

The whole process needs to be done by more than just a single nurse. Often, two nurses are involved in these steps so that they can counter-check with each other at every step they take.

Only after you're sure that the blood or blood

product is meant for your patient (by taking all the steps above or whatever steps are required by your healthcare facility), should you continue with the administration. When it's time for the administration, you must first make sure that your patient has the right venous access to receive the blood or blood product. If your patient has an existing line, you must always make sure that it's both functional and patent.

All of the aspects of blood or blood product administration must be documented including:

- All of the steps you've taken in the process of verification.

- The exact time when the infusion started and when it stopped.

- All of the information about the blood or blood product which you administered.

- All of the information about the IV line which you used for the infusion.

- The vital signs of your patient throughout the entire procedure along with the time when you recorded these vital signs.

- All of the instructions you provided to

your patient before, during, and after the administration.

When it comes to blood and blood products, there are several potential adverse reactions patients may experience. You must familiarize yourself with all of these reactions. Also, you must remember that no matter what complication or reaction your patient experiences, the first thing you need to do is stop the procedure. After this, you can start administering other intervention or care procedures.

Central Venous Access Devices

There are different types of devices for central venous access and several reasons for using them. Familiarize yourself with these different types, how to use them, and how to instruct your patients regarding their purpose, how to use the devices, how to care for them, and how to maintain them. The condition of your patient and his needs will help you determine the type of central venous access device to use.

There are two main types of venous access devices namely central and peripheral. When patients have good veins and only a short-term need for intravenous access, they can use peripheral lines with different gauges. But for those who don't have good veins and a long-term need for intravenous access, they must use central venous access devices. When it comes to the care of central venous access devices, you need to use a strict sterile technique. Depending on what type of device your patient uses, you may need to change the dressing between 2-7 days.

When placing a central venous access device on your patient, you would first place a tunnel catheter in his subclavian veins or one of the other central veins. Then you "tunnel" this catheter through your patient's skin until it exits somewhere on his chest. This makes the device more stable, especially for long-term use. You may also tunnel an implanted port under your patient's skin then thread the catheter into his superior vena cava. You can place this port subcutaneously and only access it when you need to.

On the other hand, you would place a peripherally inserted central catheter either below or above your patient's antecubital area on his non-dominant hand. Then you advance the catheter through your patient's vein until the very tip touches his cavoatrial junction or superior vena cava. You can leave this type of line in place for a period.

Both types of access devices require a sterile technique when it comes to maintenance and care. But you need to take extra precautions when caring for the central lines. Also, you must let your patients wear masks when you're performing assessments or changing the dressings. Often, you would use a chlorhexidine solution when cleaning or dressing the sites of the access devices. You must also flush the lines frequently to maintain their patency.

Dosage Calculation

For you to be able to measure and dose your patients' medications correctly, you must have a broad knowledge of the basic arithmetic concepts as well as the method of ratio and proportion when dosing medications which are in the form of a solution. It's important to note that there are different systems for measurement such as the metric system, the apothecary system, and so on, and you're likely to encounter all of them. Also, keep in mind that for the same type of medication, the dosages of adults and children or infants will vary. So you must familiarize yourself with all dosage calculations for you to correctly administer the medications to your patients.

Most of the time, you would have to base the medication dosages on the body weight of your patients. After taking the weight of your patient in kilograms, take the cc/ml/mg of the medication then multiply the two values together. The result is the total daily dose to give to your patient. After finding out the proper dosage, it's time to find out the medication dosing schedule. When figuring this out, divide the value of the total daily dose by how many times a day the medication must be administered.

For IV fluids, you have to perform a calculation to determine the rate of delivery to give to your patient. For this calculation, take the total volume of the solution and divide this by the total time of minutes you should administer all of it. Then, multiply the value by the drip/drop rate of the IV tubing you will use.

Apart from performing the required calculation, you also need to utilize your critical thinking skills when making decisions. Although errors in calculations are unavoidable, it's important for you to critically and carefully assess your answers. Ask yourself whether the answers you came up with make sense while thinking of your patient and the information you have about the drug.

Expected Actions and Outcomes

It's also your responsibility to think about the expected actions of and the intended outcomes for any medications you administer to your patient no matter how you gave it. Yes, this is a daunting task, but the good news is that there are several resources and tools which you can use to help. Learn about all of these and start using them regularly.

When you're learning about the medication prescribed for your patient, you can consult with a reference source that's factual and trustworthy. A good place for you to start is the formulary of your healthcare facility. You may also ask about the medication from the pharmacist in your facility. Other helpful resources are online websites (make sure they're reliable), a Physician's Desk Reference or PDR, and Nursing Handbooks.

Another aspect you must be aware of is all of the medications your patients are currently taking, how well they're complying with their medication regimens, and if they're experiencing the expected effects of those medications. You also have to observe and evaluate your patients for any side effects, adverse effects, toxicity or interactions from the medications they're taking. The best thing to do is to reconcile the actual use of your patient's medications which what's written on his medical record. Do this periodically.

When it comes to clinical decision making, it's important for you to integrate all of the information you've gathered from the different sources and use that as a guide for your thought processes. It's also your job to assess and document all of the responses your patient has to a specific type of medication.

Medication Administration

Administering medication is not just about giving the drug to your patient. This process involves the development of a kind of "mental checklist" to make sure that you perform all of the required steps before, during, and after administering any medication no matter what type of drug it is. As a nurse, it's important for you to be familiar with the different types of medications, how to administer them correctly, what they're for, and so on. But it's also your responsibility to educate your patients regarding the medications they need to take for their treatment.

It's important for you to have a conversation with your patients and their family members or caregivers about all of the aspects of the medications they need to be taking. The most relevant information requires the name, dosage, purpose, any potential interactions of side effects, and instructions on how your patient must take the medication. You must also inform your patients about the proper storage and protection of the medications, how it's important to finish all of the prescribed medications, and when to consult with a healthcare provider if your patient is experiencing any issues or has any questions.

When educating patients about self-administered medications (such as injections, inhalers, and the like), teach the proper technique as well as how your patient must correctly dispose of any bio-hazardous materials or unused drugs. Before you start administering any medications to your patients, there is some important information you must review namely,"

- the "rights of administration,"

- the data of your patient, and

- the medical history of your patient.

There are several aspects involved in medication administration. First of all, you must have enough knowledge about the basic pharmacological principles which are pharmacokinetics, distribution, administration route, excretion, and metabolism. You must also understand how all of these principles apply to the medications you're administering and to your patient as well. You must also ensure that you understand how to properly prepare and administer each of the medications both to children and to adults.

There are some situations where you may have to combine two types of medications coming from different vials before injecting them into your patient. This is another procedure which you must familiarize yourself with, so you can demonstrate it and educate your patients about it when needed.

Part of medication administration is documentation. You must keep a record of the medications you've administered as well as the ones you've held, omitted, or those which your patient refused to take. Also, document the administration route of the medication (IM, oral, IV, sublingual, and so on), what you observed in your patient after administering the medications, and any therapeutic or adverse effects experienced by your patient.

No matter how careful nurses (and other healthcare professionals) are, there still exist a huge number of medical errors. Mainly, these happen because of incomplete or poor communication about the medications of patients. Therefore, it's important to perform medication reconciliation. This is a process which can help reduce medical errors greatly. In particular, this is very useful for when you admit new patients to your healthcare facility, when you transfer patients from one facility to another or when you discharge your patients. Here are some steps to follow when performing medication reconciliation:

- Make a complete list of all of your patient's current medications.

- If there are any new medications to be taken, make another list.

- Compare both lists critically and check for any inconsistencies or discrepancies.

- Document the actions you've taken and report all of your findings to the proper person (such as the patient's primary healthcare provider).

Keep in mind that all types of OTC medications, dietary or herbal supplements, vaccinations, blood, blood products, diagnostic agents, and radioactive medications must be part of the lists that you make.

Another important concept in medication administration is titration which refers to any adjustment made to the dosage of a specific type of medication based on certain criteria or parameters. Usually, these are defined in the medication order from the practitioner. The main types of medications which require titration are insulin and some types of medications for blood pressure.

Every healthcare agency or facility has its own rules and guidelines regarding the handling and the disposal of any unused medications. These include guidelines which focus on how to handle narcotics. It's very important to follow the guidelines of your healthcare institution to ensure your safety and the safety of your patients. In some cases, you may have to educate your patients in handling and disposal at home too.

Parenteral and Intravenous Therapies

You must familiarize yourself with all the basic concepts of intravenous therapy including the indications for use, the differences that exist between the fluids used as well as the equipment involved for this type of therapy. The basic types of intravenous therapies include intermittent, central, peripheral, and continuous.

As part of the preparation process, you must educate your patients about the purpose of the IV catheter, how you will place it, how your patient must care for and maintain the catheter, and any potential complications or problems your patient might encounter while using the catheter. You must also inform your patient when is the proper time to notify you about any issues. All of this information must be given to your patient before you start any IV therapy or treatment.

As a rule of thumb, the preferable vein to use is the largest vein either below or above your patient's antecubital area on his non-dominant hand. The veins in the hands or legs aren't ideal for this. Also, you must never place the IV on the same side as your patient's dialysis, paralysis or mastectomy access. It's also advisable to avoid placing the IV on veins distal to any previous access site with phlebitis or an infusion. You must always assess the condition of your patient which requires IV access when you're selecting the vein. If you need to insert large bore catheters (either for the delivery of blood products or for trauma patients), you may need to use a larger vein. On the other hand, if your patient only requires IV fluids, then you may choose the smaller veins.

There are some cases when you may have to educate your patients who need intermittent IV therapy. Your conversation must include any potential complications or issues which may arise from this kind of IV therapy. Also, talk about the specific signals or alarms which may go off on the pump equipment used and what these mean.

When it comes to preparing your patient for IV catheter insertion, it is, again important for you to educate your patient before you insert the IV catheter. During the actual insertion, make sure that you use the correct technique, especially when choosing the best vein based on the medical condition and the needs of your patient. After you've established the IV line, it's time for you to determine the proper rate of fluid or medication administration. Then observe and assess your patient's overall response to the fluid of medication along with the catheter insertion site.

Your critical thinking skills are essential when it comes to determining the drip rate needed for administering your patient's medications or fluids. Generally, you can determine the infusion rate in gtt/min by taking the total amount of medication or fluid to be given and dividing that by the number of minutes by which it should be administered. Then multiply the value you get by the drip/drop factor of the IV tubing you've used. To make this easier for you, come up with a whole system consisting of different steps which you must take before you start the process of IV catheter insertion.

Infusion pumps are widely used mainly because of their convenience. However, you must allow this device to substitute your critical thinking skills. Keep in mind that no matter how efficient infusion pumps are, they are still machines which mean that there is a possibility that they will break down or malfunction. Therefore, you must always double-check to make sure that the pump you use on your patient is functioning properly. To do this, you may have to count the drops which come out of the pump over one minute or by performing a calculation to get the total amount of IV solution which was given to your patient over a specific amount of time.

Finally, it's also essential to monitor and care for the IV insertion site. These are tasks which you must never delegate to non-licensed support staff. No matter what type of IV lines you use, these are potential infection sites which is why critical care and monitoring are required.

Pharmacological Pain Management

A lot of times, you may have patients who have a "PRN order" for pharmacological pain management. Therefore, you must have a good understanding of how to evaluate your patient to determine whether they need interventions or not. You must also understand all of the regulations associated with administering narcotic medications for pain.

When it comes to pharmacological pain management, you must familiarize yourself with using this for patients of all ages and who suffer from different types of conditions. For instance, children and pregnant women will need different methods for the management of pain. Before recommending any treatment or intervention, you must first assess your patient's level of pain. You can do this using the PQRST method, regular assessment scale for pain, and the different types of graphic or numeric scales. Also, consider your patient's vital signs as well as his non-verbal language when you're performing your pain management assessment.

The pharmacologic medications which provide an analgesic effect are broadly grouped into two categories namely non-opioid and opioid analgesics. Generally, non-opioid medications are given to those suffering from mild to moderate levels of pain while opioid medications are given to those suffering from moderate to severe levels of pain. Dosing the medications based on your patient's weight is recommended for young children, infants, and neonates. For adults, there are standard schedules for dosing. For geriatric patients, you may need to adjust their dosage if they're suffering from organ dysfunction or chronic diseases.

While performing a pain assessment, make sure to document all of your findings. Also, document the medications given, the dosage, and the medication route. Include all of this information on the medical records of your patient. Check for other documentation guidelines of your healthcare facility and follow these as well.

Because of the possibility of the illegal diversion of narcotic medications by healthcare personnel, there are strict regulatory guidelines in place which you and everyone else in your healthcare facility must follow. In most facilities, they already have an existing automated system which counts all of the narcotic medications, keeps track of anyone who accesses them, and which patients the medications are given to. In case the facility doesn't have this automated system, certain steps must be taken to prevent diversion:

- The nurse signing on a form before obtaining the narcotic medication from the pharmacy.

- Delivering a narcotic sheet along with the narcotic medication to the nurses' station.

- Placing the narcotic medication in a locked, secure container.

- Assigning a nurse to be accountable for the narcotic medication and giving her the only key to access the container. This nurse will also be responsible for counting all of the medications at the beginning and the end of her shift.

- The accountable nurse is asking for the signature of the administering nurse after she takes the narcotic medication from the storage container.

- If any of the narcotic medications need to be disposed of, two nurses must bear witness to the process and affix their signatures as proof that they attested to what occurred.

Whenever you administer any pain medication, you must observe your patients and assess whether the intended therapeutic effect is occurring on the patient. Your assessment may include using the same tools you would use during pain assessment. Then document the results on the medical records of your patient. Also, document your patient's ability to reach all of the expected outcomes as a result of the pain reduction.

Total Parenteral Nutrition

Total Parenteral Nutrition or TPN can also be called hyperalimentation. This is a type of nutrition provided to patients intravenously which bypasses his entire GI system. Although TPN is more expensive than enteral nutrition, it's required for certain patients. Of course, it also comes with some potential side effects and risk factors. You must familiarize yourself with all of these along with the basic concepts related to TPN.

It's important to be aware of, identify, and appropriately intervene if any complication or side effects occur after you administer TPN. Commonly, this nutrition is administered to patients through a central line. This comes with a risk of adverse reaction, especially when the line is improperly placed. Conditions such as hydrothorax, hemothorax, and pneumothorax may potentially occur so you must be familiar with all of their symptoms. Other adverse effects which might occur and which you must be familiar with include fluid overload, air emboli, infection, hypoglycemia, and hyperglycemia.

You must provide the proper education for all your patients on why they may require TPN and how you will deliver it. You must inform your patients of all the potential complications and risks of TPN therapy. Also, it's important to help your patients understand all of the aspects of care, maintenance, and placement of the IV line which you will use to deliver the TPN.

There are specific nursing skills which you must know and use when you're considering TPN or caring for a patient who you're giving TPN to. These skills include:

- **Assessment** which refers to verifying the patient's need for TPN and recording any baseline findings of your patient.

- **Nursing diagnoses** both potential and actual.

- **Planning** which refers to establishing your patient's expected outcomes and goals for TPN therapy.

- **Assessing the treatment response** which refers to reassessing the same criteria assessed before TPN and determining the treatment effectiveness.

The other applicable skills needed include using the aseptic technique; proper changing and maintaining the bags, bottles, and tubings;

maintaining the insertion site of the catheter; and using the proper mathematical skills to calculate and to control the infusion rate. It's also essential for you to apply your knowledge of the pathophysiology of your patient in order to avoid infection and achieve everything you need to for your patient.

When you are administering TPN, you must follow the strict sterile procedure. To prevent the formation of an air embolus is to show your patient how to perform a Valsalva procedure when changing the bottle, bag or tubing. Also, make sure to remind your patient to move quickly while performing this procedure. Assessing the response of your patient to TPN is essential as you must check for any potential complications and side effects of the treatments which you have discussed with your patient before administration.

Chapter 6: Category Review Guide for Physiological Adaptation

There are different reasons why electrolyte and fluid imbalances happen. For instance, when a patient suffers from vomiting or diarrhea, this can cause a significant drop in his levels of potassium. This happens naturally whenever patients experience either emesis or diarrhea. When this happens, it's important for you to replete your patient's potassium levels as this mineral is vital in the functions of the cardiovascular system.

Dehydrated patients may have elevated levels of creatinine and BUN are indicators of injuries involving the functions of the kidneys. The good news is that hydrating your patient may help correct these injuries. Such injuries are considered pre-renal failure since there is no direct injury to the patient's kidney. However, there is a problem with how your patient's blood flows to his kidney.

This is just one example of the importance of physiological adaptation. Often, patients would require some physiological adaptation to maintain the integrity of their physiology as much as possible. Such situations involve providing the appropriate type of care for your patients who suffer from life-threatening, acute or chronic medical conditions.

Basic Concepts Covered in Physiological Adaptation

It's important for you to promote your patient's physiological adaptation. The best way for you to do this is to manage your patient's care plan and provide the appropriate care for any patients who suffer from life-threatening, chronic or acute medical conditions. This category accounts for 14% of the total questions on the NCLEX-RN.

Body System Alterations

The body of a patient undergoes several changes in response to diseases, disease processes, interventions or surgery. Not only should you recognize these changes, but you must also know how to provide the appropriate care to your patients to help bring him back to a "normal" state of health. It's also your responsibility you educate your patient about the different changes that happen in the body of your patient and the specific care which is performed for these changes.

The care of each patient starts with your assessment of his psychological and physical health status, not just the changes which occur in his body. You must also assess your patient's ability to cope with his health situation and adapt to the changed state of impairment which, in some cases, is permanent. The assessment of your patient may also involve learning about the entire support system of your patient. Here are the concepts you must know in terms of body system alterations:

- **Drainage Tubes**

You must always monitor any drainage tube closely. It's important to check for any changes in consistency, drainage amount, color, and other significant characteristics. This may include respiratory secretions, surgical wound drains, negative pressure wound therapy, and chest tube drainage. Make yourself familiar with the proper care in the monitoring of all these.

- **Hypothermia and Hyperthermia**

You must have a good understanding of all the risk factors for the development of these conditions along with all of their signs and symptoms. Be aware of the clinical parameters which define them and the appropriate interventions to perform such as cooling, using wet packs, and hydration for hyperthermia or applying warm fluids, warming packs or a warming blanket for hypothermia.

- **Increased Intracranial Pressure**

Also, familiarize yourself with the etiology, symptoms, diagnosis, care, and monitoring of patients who have increased intracranial pressure. This includes all of the non-invasive and invasive monitoring. Also, familiarize yourself with the proper treatments for this condition depending on the severity and the underlying cause.

- **Infectious Diseases**

It's also important to familiarize yourself with all of the symptoms and signs of infectious processes such as systemic signs (including chills, fatigue, GI changes, fever, etc.) and localized findings (swelling, erythema, pustule, etc.). You should have a good understanding of the common periods of incubation for different types of infections so you can link the exposure or contact history of your patient with your findings. Also, you must be aware of the different treatments performed for infectious processes and the specific interventions depending on the affected system of the body.

- **Invasive Procedures**

It's important to know your role as a nurse during any invasive procedures. Most of these procedures are performed at bedside, so it's important to have a working knowledge. You should have a good understanding of how you will identify your patient, ho you will confirm the order, collect all of the required supplies, and prepare for the invasive procedure. Then you should assist your patients and monitor them throughout the procedure and after the procedure.

You must also document the procedure properly on your patient's medical record. Some examples of invasive procedures include thoracentesis, a central line, bronchoscopy, and so on.

- **Ostomy Care**

You must also understand the proper care and the proper way to educate patients for all types of ostomies such as tracheal ostomies, enteral ostomies, and bowel diversion ostomies. It's also important for you to understand all of the techniques utilized to maintain their patency, prevent any complications, monitor the output and intake of your patients, and ensure the correct placement for proper functioning.

- **Peritoneal Dialysis**

Familiarize yourself with all of the indications for as well as the frequency requirement of peritoneal dialysis. You should know how to properly monitor your patient before, during, and after this type of dialysis. You must also be familiar with all of the common complications and the interventions to perform during the procedure. This ensures the efficiency of the treatment and the safety of your patient.

- **Phototherapy**

Familiarize yourself with the proper uses of phototherapy in both newborns and adults. You must have a good understanding of the potential complications of this procedure in treating physiologic jaundice and all of the steps you must take to minimize the risk of these complications. You must also understand the proper way of implementing the therapy based on the order of the practitioners and how to evaluate the therapeutic effectiveness.

- **Prenatal Conditions**

You must have a good understanding of how you can identify any potential prenatal problems or complications and provide the proper intervention during pregnancy, labor, and delivery. In some cases, this may also involve problems which may arise from a surgical cesarean procedure.

- **Pulmonary Care**

Familiarize yourself with all of the parts of pulmonary hygiene care from the simple techniques such as deep breathing and coughing to more complex techniques such as postural, vibration, and percussion drainage for the elimination of respiratory secretions. You must know how to make use of and educate your patents on incentive spirometry. Specifically, you should understand how to position your patients properly when performing postural drainage and the correct location and technique for vibration and percussion.

- **Radiation Therapy**

You must monitor patients who undergo radiation therapy closely and watch out for any localized and systemic side effects of the treatment. The most common kinds of adverse reactions include fatigue, alopecia, immunosuppression, damage to the mucosa and skin, and more. Also, it's important for you to familiarize yourself with the proper lifestyle changes you must discuss with your patient including precautions in terms of sunlight exposure, proper modifications in the diet, and others.

- **Seizures**

It's important for you to understand how primary seizure disorder differs from a secondary seizure disorder. You should know all of the symptoms and signs of these conditions as well as the different kinds of seizures (clonic, absence, grand mal, tonic, and so on). You must know all of your responsibilities in terms of caring for your patients when they're suffering from seizures. Also, you should know the proper postictal care along with properly documenting the occurrence of the seizure.

- **Suctioning**

You must be familiar with the correct

procedures for when you need to perform suctioning of nasal passages, oral passages, and tracheostomy or endotracheal tubes. This may also include preoxygenation before and in between the suctioning session when necessary or as indicated.

- **Ventilator Use**

You must have a good understanding of the indications for using a ventilator and all of the potential complications of use including cardiac complications, infection, alveolar overdistension, hyperventilation, hypoventilation, and so on). Although there are specialized respiratory therapists who are responsible for monitoring the patients with you, it's still important to have a broad, working knowledge of how to care for your patients who are on ventilators.

- **Wound Care**

It's important to know all of the symptoms and signs of infected wounds. You must know how to properly educate your patients for them to promote the healing of their wounds (following a proper diet, smoke cessation, and so on). You must also know the appropriate nursing interventions which promote the healing of wounds including hydration, positioning, proper wound care, dressing changes, and others. Finally, it's important to understand the proper way to monitor the drainage devices used on postoperative patients.

It's also important to familiarize yourself with all of the principles involved with your patient's post-operative care. It's important to understand the common complications which may occur after an operation, how you can monitor them effectively, and how to intervene as needed. You should also know the proper way of removing staples or sutures.

Nursing care always involves an assessment or an evaluation of how your patient responds to any therapeutic intervention or treatment. Part of your responsibility is to assess the progress of your patient toward achieving his health goals. When performing the evaluation process, follow these steps:

- Collecting the data about your patient's current health status.

- Analyzing the data.

- Comparing the analyzed data to the expected outcome of your patient.

- Determine the failure or success of the interventions performed using your professional judgment and critical thinking skills.

- Decide whether you must continue your patient's specific care plan, discontinue it or make modifications to it depending on its effectiveness.

Finally, it's also important to educate your patients in terms of promoting his progress toward a normal state of health. Consider all of the extrinsic and intrinsic factors which can either hinder or help your patient's progress. Patient education is crucial to maximize the strengths of your patients and minimize their weaknesses to improve their overall health and outcome.

Fluids and Electrolytes

It's important to employ the proper nursing care when it comes to the fluid and electrolyte balance of your patients. It's important for you to recognize all of the signs and symptoms associated with a deficiency or an excess of important electrolytes and fluids. It's also important for you to know the most likely causes of these imbalances considering your patient's current state of health. Finally, you must know how to deal with these imbalances.

The excess of body fluids (or plasma) is known as hypervolemia. There are different factors which may cause this condition such as an inability to effectively clear excessive supplementation or fluid, an increase in the patient's sodium level or organ failure. Patients who suffer from this condition may experience tachycardia, hypertension, shortness of breath, distended jugular veins, and peripheral edema. When you perform an examination, you may also discover adventitious breath sounds and a bounding pulse.

On the other hand, a deficit of body fluids is known as hypovolemia. This may happen because of dehydration, diarrhea, vomiting or a hemorrhage. The clinical symptoms of this condition include a decrease in the patient's cardiac output, hypovolemic shock, metabolic acidosis, a multisystem organ failure, a coma or, in worst cases, death.

Our bodies have some electrolytes, and it's important to keep these levels balanced to ensure the health of your patient. Here are the different electrolytes along with the conditions which may occur when there is an excess or a deficiency in patients:

- **Calcium**

The body's endocrine feedback system is responsible for the regulation of calcium. You must have a good understanding of the most likely manifestations and causes of hypocalcemia (calcium deficit) and hypercalcemia (excess calcium). It's also important to know the common medications which may trigger an imbalance in the body's calcium levels including corticosteroids, lithium, thiazides, phenobarbital, and more. You must have the ability to recognize all of the clinical symptoms associated with hypocalcemia and hypercalcemia.

- **Chloride**

You must have a good understanding of the primary metabolic causes of hypochloremia (low levels of chlorine) namely respiratory acidosis, metabolic alkalosis, hyponatremia, and more, and the disease processes which may produce the deficit (such as cystic fibrosis and others). You must also be able to identify the clinical symptoms of hypochloremia.

On the other hand, hyperchloremia (high levels of chlorine) can be caused by different disease processes such as diabetes, renal disease, hyperparathyroidism, and more, or through the loss of fluids due to diuresis, diarrhea or dehydration. You must also be able to identify the clinical symptoms of hyperchloremia.

- **Magnesium**

You must have a good understanding of the underlying disease and endocrine processes which have an effect on the body's magnesium levels as well as the medications which have the potential of triggering hypomagnesemia (like antibiotics, diuretics, PPIs, and so on) or hypermagnesemia (like laxatives and antacids). You must also know all of the clinical manifestations of both low and high levels of magnesium.

- **Phosphate**

You must have a good understanding of all the medications, endocrine dysfunctions, and disease processes which trigger imbalances in phosphate levels. You must also be aware of the clinical manifestations of hypophosphatemia and hyperphosphatemia.

- **Potassium**

You must have a good understanding of the most likely manifestations and causes of hypokalemia (potassium deficit) and hyperkalemia (excess potassium). It's also important to understand how potassium levels affect neuromuscular and cardiac functions.

- **Sodium**

You must have a good understanding of the most likely manifestations and causes of hyponatremia (sodium deficit) and hypernatremia (excess sodium). It's important to understand that sodium levels have a direct inverse relationship to the fluids in the body. There are several endocrine disorders which manifest with imbalances in sodium levels namely inappropriate anti-diuretic hormone syndrome, diabetes insipidus, and more.

When your patient has either an electrolyte or a fluid imbalance, you must carefully consider and try to anticipate the possible pathophysiologic responses to your patient's condition along with each of their treatments. Apart from recognizing all of the clinical symptoms, it's also important to know all of the risk factors associated with the development of these conditions. This is part of your overall evaluation of your patient.

When it comes to treating patients who suffer from hypervolemia, you may have to administer diuretic medications and restrict the patient's sodium or fluid intake to clear any excess fluid. For hypovolemia, the treatment focuses on correcting the underlying cause of the condition, and this depends on the severity of your patient's condition. Treatment options range from simple IV fluid supplementation to plasma expanders, proper positioning of the patient, and administering blood or blood products.

When caring for patients with electrolyte imbalances, you must focus on correcting the underlying cause of the imbalance. Also, you have to replace your patient's depleted electrolytes as needed or deplete any excess when applicable. There are some care management situations which may also involve emergent interventions so you must also familiarize yourself with all of these.

An important part of treatment is the evaluation of its effectiveness and safety. This includes monitoring the clinical symptoms of your patients, checking for any symptoms of electrolyte or fluid normalization, and checking for under or over-correction. In some cases, you may even have to suggest specific lifestyle modifications to your patients for maintenance in the long-term.

Hemodynamics

Caring for patients who need hemodynamic monitoring is a very complicated task. You must be able to understand the distinct changes in the pathophysiology of each of your patients along with the basic care practices for your patients who need routine or advanced hemodynamic intervention and monitoring.

It's important for you to have a good understanding of the following physiological principle:

·   cardiac output = SV x HR, where SV refers to stroke volume and HR refers to heart rate.

Your patient must have a cardiac output of 4 L/min to 8 L/min, the normal value which is needed to meet all of the physiological demands of the body. If your patient doesn't reach this value, a mild to severe impairment occurs. You must familiarize yourself with the clinical symptoms of a reduced cardiac output including hypoxia, reduced perfusion of the tissues/organs, and reduced peripheral pulses.

It's essential for you to be able to read cardiac rhythm strips properly and identify any abnormalities timely identification as well as intervention in case you detect any any potentially fatal arrhythmias. You must know all of the steps to follow when reading these strips along with the correct timings for all the waveforms, complexes, and intervals.

You must also have a good understanding of how to properly interpret sinus rhythm abnormalities (such as bradycardia, tachycardia, and others), atrial arrhythmias (atrial fibrillation, premature atrial complexes/contractions, atrial flutter, and supraventricular tachycardia), and ventricular arrhythmias (ventricular tachycardia, Torsades de Pointes, idioventricular rhythm, ventricular fibrillation, asystole, agonal rhythm, and premature ventricular contractions. Also, you must have the ability to recognize the different kinds of heart block namely first, second-type I, second-type II, third degree, and bundle branch.

It's also important for you to recognize the common physical symptoms and signs of cardiac abnormalities and be able to correlate these with your EKG findings. Also, you must know how to describe the changes in the path of the electrical impulses or cardiac depolarization from what's normal then again, correlate the information with the EKG findings. You must be able to understand and differentiate between benign arrhythmias and those which are potentially life-threatening.

As a nurse, you must undergo specialized training to care for patients who are changing in their hemodynamics. However, even nurses who haven't had this specialized training must possess basic knowledge of all the principles related to cardiac care. Patients who have reduced cardiac output require both psychological and physical modifications for them to cope with the condition. Help your patients by providing them with the right strategies for diet, rest, activity modification, and pain modification as well as the different ways on how they can deal with emotional or cognitive changes which happen as a result of their reduced cardiac functions. Patients may also benefit from proper planning for risk reduction and safety because of their condition.

Familiarize yourself with the new protocols of the interventions for the different types of cardiac emergencies, and you must also have the ability to initiate all of these interventions. Also, you must have familiarity with how to monitor and maintain cardiac defibrillators/pacemakers for patients who suffer from chronic cardiac arrhythmias. When you care for patients whose pacemakers have just been placed, familiarize yourself with the common complications of the procedure. In some cases, cardiac patients need special management and care depending on their specific condition or care plan. These include:

- **Alteration in tissue perfusion, hemostasis, and hemodynamics**

You must have a good understanding and ability to recognize your patients with a reduced function of their peripheral, cardiac, and cerebral organs/tissues. You must know how to identify the symptoms and signs for each of these and correctly intervene as needed. The goal for the care of patients who suffer from these conditions is to treat and to correct any underlying cause which has been identified and encourage good tissue perfusion.

- **Arterial Lines**

Familiarize yourself with the common vessels utilized for when arterial lines are surgically placed, their purpose, and even their contraindications. You must also know the proper way to monitor your patients for the common complications caused by these devices.

- **Hemodialysis**

You must have a good understanding of the different kinds of venous access which can be used for these types of patients as well as the care that they need. You must also monitor your patients properly before, during, and after the therapy.

- **Pacing Device**

Familiarize yourself with the different types of external devices for cardiac pacing (such as transvenous, transcutaneous, epicardial, and others) as well as their indications. You must also have an awareness of the most common problems which may occur with the use of these devices and how to correctly troubleshoot or intervene if the devices work improperly or fail.

- **Telemetry**

As a nurse, you can care for your patients who are on telemetry devices or a specially trained technician may help you with their care. It's your responsibility to analyze, interpret, and intervene based on the reading of the device.

Illness Management

When it comes to illness management, nursing care typically involves more than just "providing" your patient with care. You must come up with a comprehensive plan for the management of your patient's illnesses. Such a plan includes these tasks which will help your patients manage their recovery better:

- **Continuity of Care**

As a nurse, you are the most important provider of continuity of care throughout the condition or illness of your patient. You must know how to properly provide effective, efficient, and seamless care to meet the changing and ongoing needs of your patient. This includes the coordination of care, ongoing follow-up, education, identification of the community resources, and the continuous re-evaluation and modification of your patient's care plan.

In some cases, this may also extend to nurses in charge of emergency care who are tasked to assist their patients in understanding the most important information about their condition, the signs of complications, and the proper follow-up.

- **Data Reporting**

You must have a good understanding of which patient data you need to report to his managing practitioner right away as well as the data which isn't urgent. The important data which needs reporting includes any complications or adverse reactions experienced by your patient after taking specific medications or undergoing any treatment. It's also important to report any unexpected responses or outcomes or any significant changes in your patient's condition/status.

- **Gastric Lavage**

Part of your responsibility is to perform gastric lavage if needed. When your patient requires this procedure, you must know how to perform it correctly.

- **Interventions**

It's also important for you to understand that patient recovery involves both extrinsic and intrinsic factors. Consider these factors when you're thinking about the interventions to perform for recovery. Also, keep in mind that the wellness of your patients depends on different aspects including behavioral, biological, sociocultural, psychological, environmental, and healthcare adequacy. All of these affect your patient's recovery.

- **Pathophysiology Application**

You must also have a good understanding you the pathophysiology of your patient. You must also be able to apply your understanding to your patient's illness management effectively. It's important for you to understand all of the etiologies, risk factors, clinical symptoms and signs, and all of the potential complications of your patient's condition based on your knowledge of his pathophysiology. After understanding all of this information, part of your job is to come up with an effective care plan which will prevent any setbacks in the recovery process of your patient.

- **Patient Education**

Being able to provide proper patient education is a crucial part of illness management. In doing this, you're empowering your patient. Educating your patients also guides them to make informed decisions about their care and their health. Patient education begins with your evaluation of your patient's deficiencies, needs, and health goals. Then you need to come up with the appropriate education activities which you will also have to implement based on all the information you have. Patient education may also include the caregivers or family members of your patient.

You must also familiarize yourself with care plans for patients with terminal or lifelong illnesses. You must educate them in terms of self-care, modifiable risk factors, and more. Such patients have specific education needs which differ from patients who have treatable or temporary conditions.

- **Ventilation or Oxygenation**

Patients who suffer from impaired ventilation or oxygenation need a special kind of nursing management. You must familiarize yourself with the different types of indices measured by arterial blood gas. Also, you must be familiar with procedures such as spirometry, pulse oximetry, and pulmonary function testing. Remember that your patients will need care from an entire healthcare team from different medical disciplines.

Just like with the other types of nursing care, it's important for you to assess the effectiveness of your plan for illness management. You must also be able to determine whether your patient is meeting all of the expected outcomes to reach his health goals.

Medical Emergencies

As a nurse, you play an important role, especially when it comes to medical emergencies. At a minimum, your knowledge must include:

- **Application of your knowledge and skills**

When dealing with a patient who is experiencing a medical emergency, you must be aware of the most effective intervention method. This involves a rapid assessment of your patient and being able to think about the appropriate interventions quickly. Also, keep in mind that the status of your patient may change unpredictably and rapidly.

- **Emergency care**

The other parts of emergency care you must familiarize yourself with include respiratory support, using an automatic defibrillator, advanced procedures, and protocols for cardiac life support, and the steps you must take in case an emergent wound disruption occurs.

- **Notification**

Often, you are the first member of the

healthcare team who will notify your patient's healthcare provider if your patient experiences any unexpected responses or emergencies.

- **Nursing procedures**

There are specific nursing procedures which must be followed during medical emergencies, and these depend on the condition being treated. Generally, these procedures are prioritized by airway, breathing, and circulation or ABCs. There are several medical conditions which might predispose your patient to a medical emergency which involves the different systems of their bodies.

- **Pathophysiology**

Knowing the pathophysiology of your patient is crucial in emergencies. You must find out as much as you possibly can about the past medical history of your patient as well as his current medical status. This information will help you determine the best type of intervention to perform. Also, knowing your patient's pathophysiology can help you better predict the possibility of inducing a medical emergency inadvertently during a procedure or treatment.

- **Patient education**

Although medical emergencies aren't part of typical patient education, you must try your best to keep your patients reassured and educate them regarding the situations they're in, their health status, and any interventions you're planning.

- **Psychomotor skills**

These skills may vary during medical emergencies based on the needs of your patients. Generally, though, you must know the proper way to perform CPR, evaluate and clear an airway which is blocked, and perform the Heimlich maneuver. All of these establish your patient's airway to maintain his breathing and circulation.

When it comes to emergency treatments or interventions, you are responsible for assessing and documenting all of the significant events which happened along with the responses of your patients.

Pathophysiology

Your patient's pathophysiology is very important, and this cannot be overstated. Therefore, you must have a very good understanding of this as well as the proper treatment and care of your patients who suffer from chronic or acute conditions. It's important for you to correlate all of the clinical symptoms, signs, potential risk factors, diagnostic findings, unexpected outcomes, and complications for any pathophysiologic disorder.

Furthermore, there are some of general pathophysiology principles you must understand. These include the:

- Four stages of infection;

- Five stages of infection;

- Four phases of bacterial growth; and

- Six stages of viral growth.

Familiarize yourself with the phases of wound healing as well as those of the inflammatory process. It's important for you to understand the adaptive and innate immune responses and when these happen in the disease process. Also, you must have a good understanding of the principles of passive and active immunity.

Response to Therapies

Most of the time, the response of patients to therapy is both expected and predictable. But some patients might have unexpected responses to different therapies. You should know all of the potential complications, adverse reactions, and risks of the different therapies, procedures, and interventions given to patients. You must know how to differentiate between common but undesirable events and accidental or inadvertent adverse responses.

You must have the ability to recognize the clinical signs and symptoms of both unexpected and expected complications. Understand all of the risk factors which increase the likelihood of these complications and when is the right time to intervene when you're caring for patients who have undergone any procedure, therapy or intervention including for emergency care.

If your patient suffers from any complication, you must be able to identify what it is and provide the proper nursing care to promote the recovery of your patient. As a nurse, your role in the process of recovery after a complication is the same as the process of recovery from the initial medical condition.

Chapter 7: Category Review Guide for Psychosocial Integrity

The psychosocial integrity of patients is one of their basic health needs. This refers to a state of sociological and psychological homeostasis which might get affected when a patient suffers from any crisis, stress or illness. Also, anything that threatens a person's mental, social, and emotional well-being may also disrupt his homeostasis. When you're caring for patients who have psychosocial needs, you must have the ability to anticipate, recognize, and evaluate the possible responses of your patients.

Patients who are mentally prepared and emotionally balanced will be able to cope better with their illnesses. It's even better if they have a strong support system. Such people are better equipped to deal with the challenges that come with illnesses. A lot of patients may also be able to cope well when they have some spiritual affiliation. This is because believing in a higher power and placing their hope in this higher power can be very comforting. This is also one of the reasons why a lot of healthcare facilities have their chaplaincy services which they offer to patients who need spiritual support.

Patients whose psychosocial integrity have been thrown out of balance may demonstrate different emotional responses through some coping mechanisms. Some patients may be in denial and, therefore, would refuse to accept their doctor's terminal diagnosis. Some patients may displace their frustration and anger either by behaving rudely or acting out to their nurse. Still, others may compensate for their condition by trying to improve their health in other ways such as by taking additional supplements of vitamins. All of these are normal responses and, as a nurse, you will be dealing with different types of patients who are trying to cope with their illnesses.

Basic Concepts Covered in Psychosocial Integrity

Your responsibility is to provide and direct nursing care which focuses on your patient's psychosocial integrity. You must be able to encourage and support your patient's mental, social, and emotional well-being, especially those who are experiencing a lot of stress because of their condition. In the NCLEX-RN, this category accounts for 9% of the total questions.

Abuse and Neglect

Both abuse and neglect may come in different forms. Abuse can either be emotional, physical or sexual. Neglect, on the other hand, is a type of abuse which manifests in emotional and physical ways. The one thing they have in common is that they can both affect people of all ages.

If you have a child patient and you suspect child abuse, you must report this to the appropriate government agency or the authorities. For adults and other types of patients, you must first know the laws of your state which mandate how and when to report any suspected or known cases of neglect and abuse. If the law of your state requires you to report such cases, it's important to do so and to document all of your observations in the chart of your patient. It's important that you record all of your observations objectively and clearly in your patient's medical records since these might be needed for legal proceedings.

It's important for you to stay alert and aware to recognize any of the potential abuse and neglect patients. To do this more efficiently, you must familiarize yourself with the risk factors to look out for. These include:

- **Child abuse**
    - previous or current spousal abuse
    - parental stress perception
    - major life changes within the family
    - mother is at a young age when she gave birth to the child
    - low level of education
    - minimal or absence of prenatal care
    - not having a phone or having an unlisted telephone number
    - unemployment or low income
    - physical evidence of harsh punishment or discipline

- **Domestic abuse**
  - left or planning to leave an abusive relationship
  - history of a relationship that's abusive
  - unemployed, poor or living in poor conditions
  - divorce or separation
  - history of abuse in the past
  - physical or mental disabilities
  - social isolation
  - poor support system
  - witnessed domestic violence in the past
  - unplanned pregnancy
  - below 30 years of age
  - being stalked by one's partner
- **Elder abuse**
  - Although this type of abuse can occur with both men and women, it's more common in the latter.

- This commonly occurs with elders who have any mental or physical impairment and depend on a caregiver for their daily care.

When you're working with a patient with either a known or suspected case of abuse, it's important for you to encourage communication allowing your patients to share their issues. When it comes to neglect and abuse, patient educate them is important as well as teaching them to learn more about what they're experiencing outside of the healthcare facility. Provide your patients with support, counseling, and helpful strategies which they can use to cope with their situation. Also, you may be part of the team which plans the interventions for such patients.

Behavioral Interventions

You must be able to recognize, understand, and to plan the right type of care for your patients who are experiencing any adverse psychological effects from diseases, illnesses, stress, and other problems. Intervention is crucial if your patient isn't able to properly deal with reality. Therefore, your care plan must be focused on doing everything that's needed to maintain this ability. Before you can decide the intervention, you must first be able to recognize the common indications of alterations in your patient's mental processes. These include:

- disorientation;

- changes in behavioral patterns;

- changes in sleeping patterns;

- changes in the perception of the surroundings

- inability to perform basic activities for self-care; and

- mood changes.

When it's time to create a care plan for your patient, you must customize it according to his specific needs. Make sure to focus on your patient's safety, the structure of the plan, and the management or relief of symptoms needed by your patient. While implementing the plan, you must also assess the response of your patient and make changes or adjustments as needed. When it comes to planning interventions for your patient, consider the following:

- **Group therapy**

In some patients, group therapy can be very effective. Talk to your patient about this type of therapy and, if you think it's appropriate, encourage your patient to attend a couple of sessions. If your patient doesn't respond much at the beginning, keep encouraging him until he warms up to the idea.

- **Interaction**

It's important for you to encourage your patient to maintain his normal activities and interactions each day. The normalcy will help your patient develop behaviors which are more structured and routine-based which, in turn, will help him maintain his functioning. This interaction will also provide your patient with a much-needed sense of purpose.

- **Observation**

As your patient performs his daily activities and interactions, make sure to observe him closely, especially in terms of his responses, attitudes, and behaviors. You must assess and record all of your patients' reactions to your care plan as this will help you determine which parts are working and which parts need to be adjusted.

- **Patient orientation**

In your plan, you must always include ways to help orient your patient to reality. You must also encourage your patient's caregivers, family members, friends, and the other people around him to follow suit.

- **Patient responsibility**

It's important to keep on encouraging your patients to accept responsibility for their behaviors and actions. As you do this, you must also remind them that you're always there to guide and support them as needed. If you have a good relationship with your patient, this may happen naturally.

- **Positive reinforcement**

Acknowledge the achievements of your patients and praise them for these too. If your patient experiences any failures, discuss these with them and try to analyze the failures together. This lets your patients know that you're genuinely involved in their care. It's also helpful to provide support and accountability throughout the process of treatment.

- **Patient self-control**

Self-control is very important so you must

teach your patients how to achieve self-control and maintain it. For instance, if your patient feels anxious and acts out because of this feeling, provide him with effective strategies which he can employ to be able to control himself.

• Relationship

When working with your patient, you must always maintain an honest and open relationship. From the start, you must verbalize all of your expectations. This will help your patient understand his health goals and work with you to meet them.

• Role-modeling

Whenever you're working with a patient, you must always be a good role model, especially when it comes to interacting and behaving towards other staff members and patients. This demonstration will help your patients understand what you expect of them. It also supports and reinforces the information you shared with them about behavior expectations.

• Verbalizing

Even if your patient performs any inappropriate behaviors, you must verbalize your acceptance of him. Doing this will strengthen your relationship as well as your patient's trust in you. This will also remind your patient that you're there for him and you want him to meet all of his health goals.

Dependencies

Any addiction might become an impairment in the ability of your patient to properly function. But the sad news is that addictions are very common. It can be very difficult to treat a patient dealing with psychological or physical dependencies effectively.

One of the most common types of dependencies is known as substance use disorder. This refers to a person's recurrent use of substances such as drugs or alcohol. The excessive use of these substances causes a functional or clinical impairment in the person which soon manifests as physical disabilities, chronic medical problems or even an inability to perform his responsibilities at home, at school or work. Depending on the number of diagnostic criteria the patient meets, this disorder may be classified as mild, moderate or severe. The criteria are social impairment, pharmacological criteria, performing risky behaviors, and evidence of losing control.

Apart from substance abuse disorder, some patients may also have a dependency on other things such as sex, pornography, gambling, and more. All of these fall under "non-substance-related disorders" but treating patients who suffer from these is similar to the treatment of substance abuse.

As a patient, you have an important role in the treatment of your patient in terms of providing the support needed for:

- **Family and friend education**

Patients who are recovering from dependencies require a strong support system to ensure the success of their treatment. You can help your patient's family and friends learn the different ways of encouragement and support.

- **Intervention**

Part of your responsibility is to encourage and support your patients so that they stick with the different intervention procedures such as group therapy and counseling.

- **Patient education**

You will serve as a valuable educational resource which means that you should be able to provide your patients with information about the potential social, occupational, and health dangers of dependency.

- **Patient safety**

The physical symptoms that patients experience because of withdrawal can be both difficult and painful. In some cases, you have to use physical restraints on your patients to ensure their safety.

- **Physiological stability**

Provide your patient with relief from the physical symptoms they're experiencing from toxicity or withdrawal. Of course, you need to make sure that you only perform the appropriate measures for the relief of your patients.

- **Referral and follow-up**

When your patients are in the process of recovery, you may have to refer them to outside facilities or healthcare providers. Then it's your job to follow-up regarding the health of your patient and evaluates the success of his treatment. When it comes to these processes, nurses are very much involved.

When it comes to dealing with patients with dependencies, you must always take the time to talk about the effectiveness of the care plan depending on its outcome with your patient.

Stress Management and Coping Mechanisms

Patients who have just started on a new medical treatment or procedure can feel very stressed. This ordeal can also be very stressful for their families. Each of your patients has their coping mechanisms that he will have to use as he deals with his situation and you play a very important role in this trying time. You must be able to evaluate your patient's stress level, identify his coping mechanisms, provide him with resources to learn the skills he needs to cope, and determine when your patient can cope well or not. If needed, you may also have to intervene.

For some patients, they will express how they're feeling verbally. But for others, this is saying what they feel isn't their style. Therefore, you must be able to identify the most common stress responses so you can help your patients cope with their current situation effectively. These common stress responses include:

- **Cognitive**

Sometimes, when a patient is faced with an extremely stressful situation, he may start suffering from cognitive issues. Since your patient's daily life has been disrupted, this leaves him unable to effectively process the information he receives about his environment and the situation he is in. This, in turn, may affect your patient's ability to make decisions. When planning interventions, focus on trying to help your patients organize their thoughts so that they can feel more "in control" over what they're dealing with.

- **Physical**

When a patient experiences physiological effects because of stress, these may cause an imbalance in the equilibrium of his body. When this happens, your patient may experience a natural "fight or flight" response coming from his sympathetic nervous system. Patients who have physical stress responses may have a slower recovery rate. This might even make them more susceptible to other diseases.

In particular, chronic stress might start taking its toll on your patient's organ systems causing some harmful changes. It might even cause the lymphatic system to atrophy and even cause the enlargement of the adrenal gland. In terms of interventions, you must concentrate on providing your patient with adaptive responses externally to support his recovery process.

- **Psychological**

The psychological changes which occur in patients who are experiencing high levels of stress may influence or alter their emotions. Your patients might start feeling anxious and overwhelmed with their current health situation. In some cases, patients experience drastic mood swings which they cannot control. Once the patient starts experiencing chronic stress, he might end up becoming depressed. In cases where your patient experiences psychological stress responses, your interventions must concentrate on stress reduction methods such as anger management, relaxation techniques, and others.

You must be able to help your patients learn how to reduce the adverse effects that come with stress and stressful situations. Remember that doing this may be a lot harder for others because stress affects people differently. Here are some tips which you may use to help your patients deal with stress:

- Speak to your patients about what they

believe is causing stress in their lives. Then talk about the stressors which they can change and those which they can't.

- Speak to your patients and encourage them to talk to you whenever they feel the effects of stress.

- Identify the strengths of your patients, then help them learn how to make use of those strengths and the other resources they have to deal with their stressful situation.

- Ask your patients how they've dealt with stress in the past. Find out if their coping mechanisms can be applied to their current situation.

- If your patient needs new strategies to cope, help him learn these strategies. Think about the best ways to help your patient cope and discuss these with him.

- Be a good and supportive listener to your patients. If they need to say something or they need to vent about how they're feeling, allow them to. Don't just hear them out, acknowledge what they're saying and encourage the people in their support system to do this too.

Sometimes, patients aren't able to cope with the stressful situations they are in. There are several reasons for this, and it may be helpful for you to learn them. However, it's more important for you to find ways to help your patient cope to promote his process of recovery. Here are some tips:

- Have open discussions with your patients. Encourage them to maintain open communication with you by not judging them for what they say.

- When it comes to problems with their decision-making skills, be there for your patients to guide them and to bring more normalcy to their routine.

- For those patients who are struggling, they might end up lashing out or acting out at the people around them. Some even perform self-destructive actions. For these types of patients, keep an eye out and try to extend your patience and understanding when dealing with them.

- Observe your patients to see if they start manifesting physical symptoms because of the stress they're feeling. Symptoms such as frequent headaches, GI problems, and other non-specific complaints may be indications that your patient isn't handling the stress well.

- Also, observe your patients to see if they start manifesting psychological symptoms because of the stress they're feeling. Symptoms such as erratic mood swings and general irritability are common indications that your patient isn't coping well with his stressful situation.

When you notice that your patient isn't able to cope with his stress and you're finding it difficult to help him out, you may want to find out the cause of his stress. In doing this, you may be able to come up with coping strategies or resources which will be most beneficial for your patient. The common causes of stress include:

- a diagnosis of a serious or terminal illness;

- a change in the patient's health status;

- problems with the patient's support system;

- inadequate coping mechanisms; or

- a major situational crisis.

Apart from coping mechanisms, some patients may have defense mechanisms which refer to unconscious reactions or behaviors to a stressful situation or a stressor. Again, each patient has his defense mechanism, and it's your responsibility to recognize these behaviors and determine whether they're harmful or helpful to your patient:

- **Acting out** is when your patient makes use of drastic or disruptive behaviors to express a feeling or a thought which he feels he cannot express.

- **Denial** is when your patient doesn't acknowledge a feeling or a thought.

- **Displacement** is when your patient directs his feelings or thoughts to another person.

- **Dissociation** is when your patient starts to partly detach himself from his situation in an attempt at avoiding his feelings or thoughts.

- **Intellectualization** is when your patient attempts to "rationalize" a feeling or thought so he doesn't have to deal with its emotional impact.

- **Isolation of effect** is when your

patient separates a particular feeling or thought from the rest of his feelings and thoughts.

- **Projection** is when your patient believes that other people have that same feeling or thought.

- **Suppression** is when your patient acknowledges a feeling or a thought then tries to hide or ignore it.

- **Rationalization** is when your patient tries to deny his personal feelings or thoughts then tries to adopt different explanations as justification.

- **Reaction formation** is when your patient changes how he feels or thinks to the exact opposite then starts to adopt that stance.

- **Regression** is when your patient makes use of immature reactions or behaviors to deal with his feelings or his thoughts.

- **Sublimation** is when your patient turns a negative feeling or thought into behavior which generates a positive result.

As a role, you must provide your patients with a lot of chances to express their apprehensions, feelings, and thoughts. Talk to them and help them set realistic health goals and learn effective problem-solving strategies. Also, try to come up with helpful resources for your patient. Emphasize the importance of a good support system to help your patients improve their coping skills and relieve stress.

Crisis Intervention

Anyone who experiences a sudden, impactful crisis may experience emotional distress which, in turn, may hurt his daily life. As a nurse, you may also have to assist patients who are dealing with crises. Such patients may be undergoing several emotional changes which might start taking a toll on their overall health. As a nurse, you must be able to recognize your patients who are experiencing crises. Once you've recognized these issues in your patients, there are specific tasks you must do:

- Establish your patient's history with the crisis he's experiencing by gathering all of the relevant information.

- Talk to your patient about how he's

feeling because of this crisis.

- Evaluate the access of your patient to support systems to determine whether they will be able to help him out.

- Think about the safety of your patient and provide the emotional and physical support he needs to cope with the crisis and go back to how he functioned before experiencing the crisis. If needed, teach some effective coping strategies and skills to your patient as well.

- Finally, you must also assess whether your patient has the potential to perform activities which will harm himself or other people.

After performing all of these tasks and gathering all of the information you need, you may start with your nursing evaluation and diagnosis to develop a customized and effective plan for your patient's care. Generally, your goals for your patients must be:

- The reduction of stress through effective coping strategies such as visualization, relaxation, and more.

- Come up with a solution to help your patient identify any existing support system or find new ones based on what your patient needs.

- Help your patient go back to how he used to function before he experienced the crisis and all the effects that came with it.

Cultural Awareness and Influence on Health

As a nurse, you must assess, understand, and have respect for the roles of the varying ethnic, radical, and cultural perspectives in terms of how you provide care to your patients. Culturally competent nurses can recognize the world views of their patients within the context of providing appropriate care. It's important to maintain flexibility and a willingness to use new knowledge and ideas in your plans for your patients.

Talk to your patient about their views and make sure to listen to everything that they say. Then try to learn all that you can about the beliefs of your patients on illnesses and health and do this with understanding, acceptance, and tolerance. Be open enough to incorporate into your care plan the non-traditional practices and processes of your patients.

If your patient isn't able to express himself well in a language you understand, find someone who can interpret what he's saying so that you can gather all of the information you need about the cultural preferences and practices of your patient. Then document the process you used to meet the individual language needs of your patient.

Remember that culture is an important part of a person's perception of care as well as his overall health. Therefore, you must provide the proper services and care to your patients which don't contradict his cultural beliefs. In doing this, you can improve your care quality and increase the chances of a positive outcome. Right now, this type of care is a nursing standard in our multicultural and diverse population.

As you implement your care plan with these considerations in mind, you must also assess its effectiveness with your patients. If you need an interpreter to understand the insights of your patients to make your assessment, ask help from one. This ensures that you know exactly whether your care plan is working well or not.

End of Life Care

When it comes to the end of life care, each patient has his perspective of this based on his own cultural, religious, and personal background. Therefore, you must customize your end of life care plan based upon the individual factors of each patient. Of course, your main responsibilities are the same for all patients. As a nurse, you must be impartial in relaying treatment options or any other medical information to each of your patients while providing education and support as needed.

Keep in mind that all of your patients have the right to make informed decisions in terms of treatment. They may also refuse the treatment as part of their right. Talk about the individual health goals of your patient along with his family. If your patient has any priorities or wishes, you must respect all of them not just because it's the right thing to do but also because you're ethically and legally bound to.

Part of your responsibility is to prepare and provide your patients and the members of their family with the information about what they should expect when your patient is nearing the end of his life. This includes all of the psychological, emotional, and physical changes as well as deterioration or a decline up to your patient's death. Also, you must be able to help the family of your patient to cope with the anxiety they will feel as it grows each day as the death of their loved one approaches. You must always express to your patient and his family that you and all of the members of the healthcare team are doing everything you can to make your patient feel relaxed at this time.

When one of your patients dies, you must accept the loss and express your sympathy to his loved ones. Only after you've asked the deceased's loved ones about their next step should you provide them with the chance to view the body of the deceased.

Family Dynamics

In the same way that not all patients are the same, not all families are the same either. Each family will have its weaknesses and strengths in terms of how they deal with their loved ones who are terminally ill or are suffering from different medical conditions. In an ideal world, all of the families of your patients will listen to, support, and have empathy for the one who is suffering. But the sad truth is that a lot of families these days have some form of existing dysfunctional communication. The more severe this is, the more it may lead to your patient's impairment.

There are several reasons why families become dysfunctional such as:

- genetics;

- the current developmental stages each of the members of the family is in; and

- the family's lifestyle.

You may recognize a dysfunction in the family if they don't communicate well, they have poor coping skills or mechanisms, and they don't know how to draw strength from external support systems. As a nurse, you must observe the families of your patients and evaluate them for any indications of dysfunction. If you observe any of these indications, you must incorporate them into the treatment plan of your patient. One possible intervention to suggest is family or group therapy wherein you will encourage them to participate and talk about realistic ways they can help improve the way their family functions.

Grief and Loss

When a person experiences loss, one of the first responses he would have if grief. Each person has a different way of grieving whether it be social, mental, physical, emotional, or spiritual. As a nurse, the very first thing you must do is to identify and evaluate your feelings in terms of death or dying. Do this before you try to help people with their own feeling of grief and loss.

There are varied conceptual theories and frameworks which explain the process of unresolved or complicated and normal grieving and it's important for you to be aware of these. Perhaps the most well-known of these theories and frameworks is the Stages of Grieving by Elizabeth Kubler-Ross. According to this theory, when a person is grieving, he goes through five different stages namely denial, anger, bargaining, depression, and acceptance. To be able to understand the needs and responses of your patients or their family members, you must be able to recognize the stage of grief they are in. A lot of factors have an effect on these stages and the process of grieving namely:

- gender;

- age;

- cultural influences;

- developmental stage;

- physical reserves;

- emotional reserves; and

- personal strengths.

Apart from providing your patients with psychological, emotional, and physical support, there is some legal issues you must be aware of after one of your patients dies. These include:

- **Advance directives:** You must know and respect all the dying wishes of your patient. If your patient doesn't have any advance directives, part of your responsibility is to talk about this with your patient and his family.

- **Autopsy:** Sometimes, an autopsy is legally required after a patient's death. But in some cases, the patient or a member of his family may request for it.

- **DNR orders:** These orders are also part of the advance directives. The patient should have already talked about this with his family. But if your patient didn't inform his loved ones, then it's your job to talk to them about it when the need arises.

- **Organ donation:** Whatever the patient wants to be done to his physical remains after he dies may be included in his advance directives. Again, discuss this with your patient and his family before the time comes.

There are other ways where you can provide support to your patients and their loved ones during the end of life care. These include:

- Providing your patient's loved ones with strategies for coping with the emotions they're feeling such as loneliness, fear, anxiety, and more.

- Most patients who are approaching the end of their lives may experience a loss of control over their own lives. In such cases, provide your patient with a lot of reassurance to lessen this negative feeling.

- You may also encourage your patients and their loved ones to have open discussions about how they are feeling. If you think it will help, you may suggest that they join bereavement groups or other external support systems.

- There are some measures you can take to provide your patients with physical comfort such as sedation, pain control, positioning, and so on.

- Talk to your patients about their emotional reactions and provide them with reassurances if these are normal reactions. Educate your patients about the natural process of grieving which is a healthy response to the situation they are faced with.

- Spend some time with your patients and their families during this difficult time. Listen when they need to talk or vent and provide reassurances and support to make them feel better.

Mental Health Concepts

Mental health refers to the psychological and emotional well-being of a person. If a person has good mental health, he will be able to function normally every day. A person who has good mental health will be able to act responsibly, will be aware of himself and his actions, will have a positive mood, and will be worry-free most of the time. He will also have adequate coping mechanisms and skills to help him deal with the stressors and hassles of everyday life.

There are many factors which may influence a person's mental health including:

- genetics;

- childhood nurturing;

- childhood attachment;

- life circumstances, and more.

Apart from trying to maintain good mental health, a person must also possess adequate interpersonal skills for communication, be able to use his ego defense mechanisms properly, and have access to great support systems.

As a nurse, you must be able to evaluate the mental health needs or issues of your patient. Then plan your care plan around these needs and issues. You may have to provide different types of care for just one patient. Also, you may need to use your psychopathology knowledge on your patients to provide them with the best mental health care possible.

Religious and Spiritual Influences

By definition, religion is a formalized and organized set of beliefs which are based on one god or several gods. On the other hand, spirituality refers to the "connectedness" of a person to others, to his environment, to the universe, to a higher power, and himself.

Both spirituality and religion can have huge effects on the health outcomes and the psychosocial and physical well-being of patients. Therefore, maintaining the spiritual and religious balance of your patients may help improve their overall health. To do this, you must have a good understanding of how your patient's spiritual or religious beliefs affect how they perceive and how they will react to the clinical care that you provide.

As a nurse, you must listen to your patients both empathetically and respectfully when they talk about their spiritual or religious needs. You should also make yourself aware of the various spiritual and religious traditions which are different from your own. After understanding these traditions, you must plan and provide care to your patients which is consistent with his own beliefs and values. And if a patient refuses care because it doesn't align with his spiritual or religious beliefs, you must respect that as well.

Sensory and Perceptual Alterations

These refer to the disruptions in the cognitive functions of a patient which, in turn, cause him to have a distorted perception of his environment and how he interacts with other people. When sensory and perceptual alterations occur, these might result in a patient being unable to function normally which places him in a dangerous situation. There are several precipitating factors which may affect sensory functioning of your patient namely:

- **Culture:** There are different cultures which exist in the world, and they may have varying norms for personal space, eye contact, and other forms of sensory functioning.

- **Developmental stage:** The age of your patient and any physical deterioration may affect your patient's ability to see, hear, and so on.

- **Illnesses:** There are specific conditions

and illnesses which may have a severe effect on the perceptual and sensory functioning of your patients. These illnesses may have a more critical nature such as stroke and cancer. Furthermore, chronic diseases like hypertension, diabetes, and some neurological disorders may affect your patient's ability to receive and process sensory stimuli properly.

- **Lifestyle:** Patients who have just experienced a recent lifestyle change may also start experiencing impairment in their sensory functioning.

- **Medications:** There are some types of medications such as opioids and benzodiazepines which may affect the sensory functioning of your patient. Other medications such as Lasix and gentamicin, on the other hand, may have an ototoxic effect on your patients.

- **Personality:** Some patients might experience difficulties if they are aloof, introverted, or aren't able to communicate well.

- **Stress:** Emotional and physical stressors may affect the cognition of your patient.

It's important for you to know all of the risk factors for sensory and perceptual alterations. Knowing these risk factors and being able to identify them in your patients will allow you to take the necessary preventive interventions to keep your patients safe. These risk factors include:

- **Acute illnesses:** Patients suffering from infections, high-fever, intoxication, and seizures may need proper interventions for their sensory alterations.

- **Close observation:** Patients who are closely observed or monitored like those who are in the Intensive Care Unit may start experiencing sensory alterations because of too many stimuli.

- **Discomfort and pain:** There are appropriate nursing interventions to perform for such patients such as positioning, administering medications, and more.

- **Issues with cognitive abilities:** Patients who suffer from conditions which disrupt their cognitive abilities may need specific types of interventions.

- **Emotional disorders:** There are several nursing interventions you can perform for patients with emotional disorders. Make sure to tailor these interventions to the specific needs of your patients.

- **Environment:** Patients who have very minimal sensory stimulation might start experiencing adverse cognitive effects.

- **Minimal social contact:** For these types of patients, you need to provide intervention to prevent the symptoms of sensory deprivation.

- **Problems with hearing and vision:** For such patients, you must use the proper nursing interventions such as communicating through sign language, using assistive devices, and more.

- **Restricted mobility:** Make sure that your patients who have this problem can get their personal belongings, have access to various activities, and have the help they need to move when they need to.

Support Systems

Support systems are crucial for any patient. They need their support system to provide them with practical, moral or emotional support as needed. The support systems of your patients may help them with their process of recovery. These support systems may also help educate your patients so they can better understand the condition they're suffering from as well as the treatments they need to overcome their condition.

Although nurses and the other members of a patient's healthcare team take care of patients in valuable ways, support systems may provide help in different ways. For instance, family members may help your patients learn the skills they need to care for themselves better. These people may also help patients maintain the lifestyle changes they need for the treatment of their condition.

As a nurse, you have to work hand-in-hand with your patient's support system. This may involve helping the family members or the caregivers of your patient by giving them access to any external resources they may need to help your patients.

Therapeutic Communication

Therapeutic communication involves more than just having discussions with your patient. This process involves interaction, planning, and goals which are specifically tailored for your patients. Therapeutic communication aims to provide your patient with a place to have open and constructive communication. To do this, you must form a beneficial and positive relationship with your patients which is based on trust.

This type of communication involves you listening to your patient and trying your best to understand him. The absence of therapeutic communication may lead to an impairment in your patient's process of recovery. It's important to note that part of therapeutic communication is nonverbal communication. Nonverbal communication can sometimes be more powerful than its verbal counterpart as this uncovers your patient's true attitudes and feelings. There are certain foundations you need to establish for therapeutic communication including:

- **Ability to participate:** You must always make sure that your patients can participate in the process of therapeutic communication. If not, you may have to make adjustments to the process to help your patient with his participation.

- **Causes of unsuccessful communication:** You must be able to communicate with your patients successfully. If there are any factors which are causing ineffective communication between you and your patients such as distractions, education level, language barriers, and others, make adjustments to how you communicate as needed.

- **Communication skills:** The communication skills and styles differ from one patient to another. Evaluate your patients carefully and make adjustments to your communication sessions to meet their individual needs.

- **Non-verbal communication:** Keep in mind that eye contact, body positioning, and other non-verbal, physical cues can be more powerful and effective than what your patients say.

- **Understanding the communication factors:** You must have a good understanding of the age;

developmental level; understanding and consciousness level; ability to communicate effectively; and the perspectives, perceptions, values, and culture of your patients.

If you want to have a successful therapeutic communication and therapeutic relationship with your patients, the presence of these factors is essential:

- **Appropriate confrontation** which refers to gently discussing your patient's need to deal with specific problems or issues. You must do this in the most acceptable way possible, and it's only recommended for those who have established a good relationship with the patient.

- **Empathy** refers to the sharing and understanding of another person's feelings.

- **Genuineness** which refers to expressing and showing your sincere and honest concerns for the questions and concerns of other people.

- **Respect** which refers to the regard and acceptance of other people even though they have different perspectives or beliefs.

- **Self-disclosure** which refers to your sharing of your own experiences and views to improve the emotional and mental state of the other person.

- **Specificity and concreteness** which refers to making use of direct and specific terminology when you're communicating instead of using vague or general terminologies.

Unfortunately, there are several barriers which may hinder the establishment of your therapeutic relationship. Therefore, you must try your best to avoid the following barriers:

- **Being defensive:** often, patients are defensive because they don't want you to learn about their perceived or real shortcomings or failures. You must try to get around this defense mechanism as it's not at all therapeutic for the patient.

- **Being judgmental:** your responsibility to your patient is to listen well and try your best to understand where he's coming from. It's not your job to pass judgment nor is it your job to place any value on the message your patient is trying to convey.

- **Challenging, probing, rejecting or stereotyping:** all of these are highly counterproductive and will prevent you from establishing a strong therapeutic relationship with your patients.

- **Improper decoding:** this is not being able to recognize the true and intended message your patient is trying to convey.

- **Listening issues:** these include a patient's inability to listen properly. Therefore, you must make time to communicate properly with your patients by minimizing distractions.

- **Putting your needs before your patient's:** yes, you have a lot of work to do and so little time to do it. But you must always place the needs of your patients before your own if you want to be able to listen and communicate effectively.

- **Trying to change the subject:** you must be able to identify your personal feelings about intense or difficult subjects then cope with all of them before you start communicating with your patients. It's not appropriate to try and change the subject because you feel stressed or uneasy about it.

How you respond to the feelings or thoughts you patient communications with you can go a long way in building a strong therapeutic communication. Here are some effective techniques to employ:

- **Clarification:** There are specific techniques such as restating, paraphrasing, and exploring which helps ensure your patient that you're hearing and understanding his message correctly. This also helps ensure that you don't place your assumptions or biases on what your patient is saying.

- **Reflection:** Here, you will reflect the emotions of your patient to him during your discussion. This will allow your patient to explore his feelings further and express the unspoken ones too.

- **Silence:** Simply listening to your patients without interrupting lets they know that you're thinking about what they're telling you. In most cases, silence also shows that you accept everything your patient is saying. Finally, this technique allows your patient to take the lead in the process of communication.

- **Using leads:** Starting your conversation off with a good opening statement will encourage your patient to open up to you. Using leads also tells your patient what you want to learn more about him by hearing what he has to say. This technique also allows your patient to drive the direction of your discussion.

You must provide the proper interventions and care to help your patients adapt more effectively to their environment to promote their recovery. To do this, you must meet all the needs of your patient. You must determine whether or not your patient can perform self-care activities effectively. You must also check if your patient is finding it challenging to adapt to his care environment. Provide your patient with a safe and supportive environment for his recovery. Maintaining this type of environment involves eliminating all of the avoidable and extraneous stressors.

Nursing and Psychosocial Integrity

As a nurse, you have to make use of the different nursing processes for evaluation, diagnosis, care planning, and implementation to care for and support the physiological integrity of your patients. In doing this, you show your patients that you understand, respect, and empathize with them in their time of crisis, injury or illness. Utilizing the nursing process properly also gives your patients the freedom they need to take on an active role in their care plan.

Nurses are important as they play a very important role in observing patients, using their psychopathology knowledge, and interacting with patients closely to provide help and interventions as needed. In doing this, you ensure the protection of your patient's psychosocial integrity.

Chapter 8: Category Review Guide for Reduction of Risk Potential

Even though patients go to hospitals and other healthcare facilities to get well, most types of medications, treatments, and interventions also come with the potential for risk. So the best thing you can do along with the rest of the healthcare team is to reduce this risk potential to ensure the safety of your patients. For instance, diagnostic tests are very important as you can use them to determine the condition of your patient based on the symptoms he is manifesting. However, some tests such as MRI and CT scan involve the use of contrast dyes which, unfortunately, some patients are allergic to. Therefore, you must evaluate your patient first and inquire about any allergies he has before performing such tests.

If your patient is allergic to the contrast dye

used in CT scans or MRIs, you cannot use it for the test. Also, keep in mind that MRI isn't appropriate for patients who have any metal inside their bodies such as pacemakers or tissue expanders. For patients who are allergic to contrast dyes, you may use water or barium instead. Even if you do utilize the contrast dye (after making sure that your patient isn't allergic to it), you must inform your patient that he needs to drink a lot of fluids to flush out the dye from their system because it affects the kidneys. Other types of diagnostic tests to consider are EKGs, stress tests, x-rays, and echocardiograms.

Another effective way to determine your patient's condition is to take a look at his laboratory values. For instance, if your patient is experiencing a shortness of breath, check his hemoglobin levels to see if he's suffering from anemia. Or if your patient is experiencing chest pain, check his troponin level to see if it's elevated as this may indicate a heart injury. Liver function tests, on the other hand, allow you to check your patient's liver function and such tests would be required for patients who appear jaundiced.

Surgeries also come with risks for complications. One way to prevent this is through a "timeout." This is a period before the surgical procedure begins where everyone inside the operating room stops to verify the patient, the body part of the patient they will be operating on, and the surgical procedure which is about to take place. These are some examples of steps taken to reduce the risk potential.

Basic Concepts Covered in Reduction of Risk Potential

This category refers to how you, as a nurse, would help reduce the risk of patients to experience health problems or complications because of their illnesses or the procedures and treatments they need to undergo. This category accounts for 12% of the questions on the NCLEX-RN.

Vital Signs

Knowing how to read the vital signs of your patients is a basic skill, and this is one of the quickest assessment tools, especially in terms of observing your patients for any significant changes in their physiological function and their response to your intervention procedure. Any abnormalities or changes in your patient's temperature, respiration, heart rate, oxygen saturation, and blood pressure may indicate an underlying physiologic issue.

Being able to assess your patient's vital signs is very important in determining the normal physiologic function of your patient. Since abnormalities in these physiologic functions usually come with a quick change in the patient's vital signs, you must have the ability to correlate your knowledge of the pathophysiology of your patient with any changes that occur. After observing the changes in your patient's vitals, you must perform the proper intervention as needed:

- You must know the proper way of measuring a patient's blood pressure along with the underlying physiologic functions which affect blood pressure including blood viscosity, blood volume, peripheral vascular resistance, cardiac function, and so on. You must be aware of the normal blood pressure ranges across all age groups as well as the phases of the cardiac cycles which correspond with diastolic and systolic pressures. Also, you must have a good understanding of which physiologic systems affect the blood pressure of patients such as the venous return, peripheral vascular resistance, cardiac rate, and so on.

- There are two ways to assess the pulse of your patient namely auscultation (using a stethoscope) and palpitation. It's important for you to be aware of the normal ranges and how to properly assess the pulse rate of your patients no matter what age they're in. You must also be aware of how to properly assess the apical pulse in adult patients. Take note of the regularity as well as the quality of the pulse of your patient. Also, you must know the various physiologic systems which may affect the heart rate of patients namely the parasympathetic nervous, autonomic, cardiovascular systems, and others.

- When taking your patient's respiration, you must know how to properly check for the respiration depth, quality, and rate. You must also know the normal values for different patients depending on their age. Also, you must be familiar with the various physiologic changes which may cause respiratory depression or an increase in the respiratory rate including pain, fever, alkalosis or acidosis, CNS damage or depression, and more.

- When taking your patient's temperature, you must have a good understanding of the proper procedures for checking depending on the condition and age of your patient. Also, remember that there are certain factors which may affect your patient's temperature including hormonal cycles, his emotions, and even the temperature of the environment.

All of these procedures for checking your patient's vital signs are non-invasive. However, there are also invasive methods for monitoring patients. You need to have a good understanding of the rationale and use for these invasive procedures. One such procedure is needed for the monitoring of increased intracranial pressure which is needed for patients who have intracranial bleeding, tumors, a head trauma, and more. Remember that there are plenty of symptoms which may point to an increase in your patient's intracranial pressure such as changes in the pupils, headache, a decrease in the consciousness level, vomiting, and more.

Another type of invasive monitoring procedure involves hemodynamic monitoring which may include the measurement of continuous blood pressure, central venous pressure, pulmonary artery pressure, cardiac output, pulmonary artery wedge pressure, and other indices.

Diagnostic Tests

Diagnostic tests are important for the reduction of risk potential as these tests may point to health issues which may require intervention to save your patient's life. Diagnostic tests can either be invasive or non-invasive. No matter what type of diagnostic test you're using, it's important for you to follow some general steps before you administer or assist with such tests. These steps include:

- confirmation of the order of the diagnostic test

- confirmation of the patient by using at least two identifiers which are different from each other;

- educating your patient and the members of his family about the purpose of the diagnostic test as well as any special instructions for it;

- acquiring and confirming informed consent;

- washing your hands and taking other general precautions depending on the requirements of the diagnostic test;

- labeling the specimens accurately, completely, and properly along with carefully transporting or storing the specimens;

- properly cleaning up and disposing of all of the materials collected or used during the diagnostic test, especially in terms of biohazardous waste, caustic or dangerous materials.

You must have a good knowledge base of the nursing procedures required when administering or assisting with diagnostic tests. Each of these tests has its own unique set of guidelines and procedures, and you must familiarize yourself with all of them. Also, you must have a good understanding of the purpose and the proper way to prepare for:

- cardiovascular tests including angiography, EKG, and others;

- gastrointestinal tests including barium enema, colonoscopy, and others;

- general diagnostic tests including CT scans, biopsies, ultrasound, x-ray, MRI, and others;

- integumentary tests including allergy testing, tuberculin skin test, and others;

- musculoskeletal tests including arthroscopy, bone dentistry, and others;

- neurological tests including myelography, EEG, and others;

- reproductive tests including mammogram, fetal heart monitoring, and others;

- respiratory tests including PFT, bronchoscopy, and others; and

- urinary or renal tests including IVP, cystoscopy, and others.

For most diagnostic tests, you must be able to quickly evaluate the results of your patient and compare these results with either the baseline evaluation or the results of his previous test.

This is important so that you can administer proper care to your patient. Familiarize yourself with the different testing methods which require your quick evaluation to ensure that you're prepared.

In some cases, you may have to monitor your patient's ongoing test results of the diagnostic tests such as for non-stress tests, maternal-fetal tests, ultrasound, fetal heart monitoring, and amniocentesis. Some of these tests may even need a comparison to the earlier findings from the previous tests. As soon as you discover any abnormalities in the test results of your patients, you may either perform an intervention or make modifications in the care plan of your patient. In some cases, you may also have to inform your patient's practitioner of any existing critical values which might pose immediate harm to your patient.

Laboratory Values

For you to be able to take proper care of your patient, you must have a good understanding of his laboratory values, the normal ranges of laboratory values, and the proper techniques for collection and monitoring. As a nurse, you will have to prepare your patients before they have laboratory testing. Part of the preparation is to explain to your patient the purpose of the laboratory test and any steps the patients must take to prepare themselves for the test.

Then you must also familiarize yourself with the correct techniques as well as the steps involved in the collection of blood specimens from a patient's peripheral vein and a central venous catheter. You must also know the proper way of collecting specimens from wounds, stool samples, and urine samples too.

It's virtually impossible to memorize all of the normal ranges for all of the types of specimens collected for laboratory testing. However, it will be highly beneficial for you to at least have a basic knowledge of the normal ranges for the most common laboratory tests which are ordered in your healthcare facility. These include:

- ABGs or arterial blood gasses (HCO_3, pH, PCO_2, PO_2, SaO_2);

- CBC or complete blood count (hematocrit, platelets, hemoglobin, WBC or white blood cells);

- coagulation studies (aPTT or activated partial thromboplastin time, INR or international normalized ratio, PT or prothrombin time, PTT or partial thromboplastin time)

- electrolytes (potassium, sodium, and others);

- glucose (fasting, HgbA1C or glycosylated hemoglobin, random);

- lipids (HDL or high-density lipoprotein, LDL or low-density lipoprotein, triglycerides, total cholesterol); and

- renal indices (BUN or blood urea nitrogen, creatinine).

Apart from knowing the normal ranges for the laboratory tests, you must also have the ability to critically assess the laboratory values of your patient and compare these values with his past results and with the normal values. This is important to see how well your patient is responding to the intervention or treatment. Part of your responsibility as well as to notify the ordering practitioner of your patient of any abnormalities in the laboratory values of your patient.

Body System Alterations

It's important for you to identify patients who have experienced alterations in their body systems as these can be potentially life-threatening or dangerous. In this particular area, proper nursing care plays an important role in the reduction of risk potential. There are several types of medical conditions which have the potential to place your patient at a higher risk for mortality and morbidity.

Part of your responsibility is to identify patients who have a high risk of aspiration. These include patients who are sedated, those who have difficulty swallowing, and those who are on tube feedings. Other conditions may also place patients at risk for skin breakdowns such as those who are immobile, those who have poor neurologic sensory functions, those who have urinary or fecal incontinence, and those who have a poor nutritional status. You must also familiarize yourself with the different conditions which place patients at risk for inadequate vascular perfusion including hypotension, patients with immobilized limbs, diabetes, and postoperative patients.

Although these are several conditions which cause an increase in risk, the list isn't very exhaustive. Therefore, you must be able to come up with a detailed and comprehensive nursing assessment. This will help you determine which are the potential areas which may need your nursing intervention. Familiarize yourself with the specific care and treatments to provide to patients who are at risk.

Part of your responsibility is to educate your patients about their condition and provide them with strategies for self-care. These strategies may be related to the activity level of your patients. For instance, if you have an immobile patient, you must provide education about the importance of the proper types of exercises as well as frequently changing their position to prevent the development of contractures. Also, you must educate your patients on the proper methods which will prevent any complications caused by a diagnosed illness or a disease process.

Aside from comparing the most current data of your patient with the normal data to check his progress, it's also your responsibility to monitor the data and assess for any potential side effects and complications of the therapy. Being able to monitor the data closely may help you diagnose any new conditions or illnesses which might develop during the treatment of your patient.

Complications

When a patient undergoes any procedure, test or treatment, he may be at risk for complications. In general, the more invasive the procedure, test or treatment is, the higher the risk. Therefore, you must utilize your nursing knowledge to use the proper skills to care for your patients properly. As with any medical process, assessing the patient is crucial. The assessment allows you to spot any abnormalities in the patient's response to the intervention, test or treatment. To do this, you must know all of the common potential complications. You must also look out for any subtle indications of rare abnormalities or complications.

When planning your nursing interventions, base them on your patient observations and on your knowledge of how to properly prevent complications. For instance, if your patient is on tube feeding, you must maintain the elevation of the head of his bed to just the right angle. This reduces the patient's aspiration risk. Or if one of your patient's extremities is in a cast and is immobilized, you have to perform regular assessments of the neurologic function and the circulation of your patient's limb. You must also provide patient education so your patient can observe himself for any symptoms which indicate potential complications so he can report these to you.

Another important way to prevent complications is to have a good understanding of the basic nursing care principles for patients who are at risk for these complications. For instance, you must know and use the correct aseptic technique for the care of central venous or peripheral access lines. Or you must also know that you should raise the side rails of the beds of patients who are at an increased risk for falling. Most of the time, you must apply your knowledge of the proper nursing procedures so that you can take the correct precautions.

When performing your assessment, you must concentrate on the most likely areas which might place your patient at risk for complications after undergoing any treatment, test or procedure. If your patient just had any invasive surgery or test, you must monitor him closely and frequently for any signs of bleeding, shock, and more. If your patient is using any tubing such as chest, nasogastric, and others, you may need to familiarize yourself with the proper assessment schedule of the tubing to maintain its patency. If your patient uses endotracheal tubing, you may also have to perform suctioning.

Most of the time, you will be responsible for performing specific procedures which will help reduce your patient's risk of developing complications. Some examples of procedures you may have to perform are:

- placing and removing nasogastric tubes;

- placing and removing urinary catheters;

- starting a peripheral venous access line and maintaining then removing it; and more.

You must, therefore, familiarize yourself with these procedures and more as well as when you need to perform them.

There are some special procedures which require you to take a unique set of nursing precautions to prevent any dangerous complications. One such procedure is ECT or electroconvulsive therapy. In this procedure and other similar procedures, you may have to educate your patient about all of the required considerations, implement them, then monitor your patients for any complications which might develop during and after the medical procedure.

Most of the time, you may have to provide your patient with direct intervention to avoid the development of potential complications. These direct interventions are also needed when you discover a complication upon assessment. It's important to understand all of the proper nursing interventions to avoid the development of complications to your patient's circulatory system (shock, hemorrhage, thrombosis, and so on), aspiration (foreign bodies, tube feedings, bottle feeding, swallowing disorders, and so on), any neurologic complications which may occur because of tight casts or dressings, and foot drop which occurs because of immobility.

Finally, you may also have to evaluate how your patient responded to any form of treatment or procedure. Document all of your observations from your evaluation including all of the intended effects and any complications or side effects which are unintended. You need to make use of objective data, the subjective reports of your patients as well as the findings from your evaluations, and assessments.

Patients who need to undergo surgical procedures may need special nursing care and consideration to minimize the risk of complications. Once again, there is a need for you to apply your pathophysiology knowledge when you're caring for a patient after surgery. For instance, you need to be familiar with the common symptoms of infection, pneumothorax, thrombocytopenia, hemorrhage, and the unintentional puncturing of one of the patient's major blood vessels. To know all of this, you must have a good understanding of the etiology or all potential complications and the risk factors for their development.

Nursing care after surgery starts even before the procedure. Your patients will need special instruction and education regarding the proper interventions and care after surgery to prevent any complications. Once you've implemented these nursing interventions, you must also perform the proper documentation and evaluation of these interventions.

System-Specific Assessments

You must familiarize yourself with the different types of assessments which are system-specific for your patients who have undergone treatments or procedures. You must also have a good understanding of the significance of how abnormalities affect patient healing and outcomes. This is important for you to plan the proper intervention and care.

It's important for you to know the proper way of performing and when to utilize the system-specific assessments based on different factors including:

- your patient's health status;

- the treatment or procedure underwent by your patient; and

- the potential risks associated with each of the treatments or procedures.

Here are some of the most important types of system-specific assessments:

- **Abnormal neurological status**

Assess your patient's consciousness level, the strength of his muscles, mobility, the function of his cranial nerves, and the reflexes of his deep tendons. Familiarize yourself with how to document each of these properly.

- **Abnormal peripheral pulses**

Assess your patient's major peripheral pulses then take note of how full, strong, and regular they are. Familiarize yourself with the correct rating scale to use for documentation. Also, you must know how and when to utilize the Doppler system to help with your assessment.

- **Assessment of risk**

Performing assessments and nursing diagnoses are crucial in the process of risk assessment. The findings of these assessments have a direct impact on your nursing plan. Also, these will help with your intervention planning to avoid morbidity or further illness.

- **Changes and trends in your patient's condition**

You need to make use of your ongoing assessments to monitor for any changes or trends in the condition of your patient. You must know when it's time to intervene and which type of intervention to use.

- **Factors which delay the healing of wounds**

You must know how to identify all of the potential factors which might delay or have an effect on the healing of wounds such as nutrition, alcohol or cigarette use, age, chronic health conditions, medications, and so on.

- **Focused assessment**

There are times when the health status of your patient requires a focused assessment. In such cases, you may have to perform the assessment, interpret it, and implement it too.

- **Hyperglycemia or hypoglycemia**

You must recognize and comprehend all of the clinical symptoms of both hyperglycemia and hypoglycemia including HHNS or hyperglycemic hypermuscular nonketotic syndrome and ketoacidosis.

- **Peripheral edema**

Have a good understanding of the physiological settings which lead to peripheral edema and the proper way of assessing and documenting your findings.

Therapeutic Procedures

When it comes to therapeutic procedures, your nursing knowledge is essential. Apply this knowledge for the care of your patients to reduce the risk of them experiencing any negative outcomes from their treatments. For one, it's important for you to know how to properly assess patients who are in the process of recovering from general, regional or local anesthesia as well as sedation. You must have a good understanding of these types of anesthesia and when to use them. Familiarize yourself with the risks they present and which are the tools you must use to monitor your patients who are undergoing recovery consistently. Also, you must be able to recognize any potential complications from the different types of anesthesia and when you need to perform an immediate intervention.

It's your responsibility to educate your patients regarding all of the treatments or procedures you're planning to perform. Also, you must obtain informed consent from your patient and understand when this type of consent must come from a healthcare proxy. You must also provide your patients with the proper instructions regarding self-care, post-procedure care, and the coordination of your patients home care if needed.

The nursing care that is given to your patient before the treatment or procedure ensures that he is psychologically and physically prepared to undergo the treatment or procedure. The assessment also helps you determine how appropriate the planned treatment is for the condition of your patient. During the treatment, you need to monitor the physiologic status of your patient continuously. The physical assessments also continue even after the procedure along with focal assessments which involve the organ system which has been treated.

There is a specific type of education to give to your patients who have undergone treatments or procedures. You must start with education as soon as your patient gets admitted to your healthcare facility. Patient education includes verbal discussions, learning aids, and providing specific instructions are some methods you must familiarize yourself with. Make sure to customize your patient education according to the cognitive abilities and needs of your patients.

As a nurse, you may also have to perform different types of assessments for monitoring each of your patients. For instance, if your patient has a fracture, he will require assessment of alignment, intact neurologic function, and intact circulatory function before, during, and after the cast is applied. On the other hand, if your patient underwent conscious sedation, only registered nurses with special training may administer, monitor, and care for the patient during the process of recovery. These are just some examples, and there are a lot more.

Familiarize yourself with the special kind of nursing intervention and care wherein you would take precautions against your patient's further illness or injury. This is crucial, especially when you're taking care of patients who suffer from musculoskeletal injuries. Most of the time, there are special types of assisted devices or techniques used such as an abduction pillow which prevents further injury of patients with hip fractures or the log-rolling method which helps maintain spinal alignment.

You must also know how to constantly monitor the different therapeutic devices to ensure their effective functioning. Such devices may include drainage devices for wounds, chest tubes, continuous bladder irrigation, and more. Also, familiarize yourself with the common issues associated with these devices and have a good understanding of how to determine the reason for the malfunction. Finally, you must also know when it's time to remove the device and replace it with a new one.

Chapter 9: Category Review Guide for Safety and Infection Control

This is another important category to learn when you're preparing to take the NCLEX-RN. From tasks as simple as washing your hands to those as important as preventing the spread of diseases. Here, there are some key concepts which you must be very familiar with. First of all, there are standard precautions. This is the first level in terms of infection control when caring for your patients. These precautions ensure that there is minimal risk of transmitting organisms which, in turn, ensures the safety of your patients through the control of infections.

Then there are the contact precautions which prevent the skin-to-skin transmission of diseases. Patients who suffer from skin infections such as scabies, herpes simplex, Staphylococcus, varicella zoster, and more will have these types of precautions. When dealing with these types of patients, make sure to wear the proper gear to prevent infection.

For droplet precautions, these are important for patients who are suffering from contagious illnesses such as some types of pneumonia, diphtheria, scarlet fever, and more. If you're working with patients and you need to take droplet precautions, you must place them in a private room, wear a face mask, and be aware of the safe distance away from your patient to prevent transmission. Finally, airborne precautions are those who are focused on preventing the spread of infection due to pathogens. Some of the diseases patients may suffer from are measles, chicken pox, tuberculosis, and others. Patients who suffer from such illnesses must also be placed in private rooms which have negative ventilation to prevent the spread of the pathogens. Remember to close the doors of the patient's room and wear a mask when you're providing care to the patient.

Basic Concepts Covered in Safety and Infection Control

Learning the topics in this category will help

you protect yourself, your patients, and the other members of the healthcare team from health and environmental hazards. This category accounts for 12% of the total questions on the NCLEX-RN.

Prevention

As a nurse, you play an important role in hazard prevention to patient care for accidents, medical errors, injuries, and infections. You must also have a good understanding of the various principles which ensure the safety of the healthcare staff including proper ergonomics, using all of the technology and equipment safely, and the proper handling of hazardous and infectious materials. Finally, you must also familiarize yourself with the safety factors which may affect your patients at home and your role in security emergencies and situations which require emergency responses.

When reviewing the safety issues of your patients, start with your knowledge of the developmental or age-specific risks that come with these different age groups:

- **Babies or infants**

You must provide the proper education to parents or the primary caretakers of babies or infants. Inform them that it's their responsibility to take the necessary precautions to avoid accidents or injuries. Give them reminders such as placing a baby or infant on his back after he eats or when it's time to sleep. Also, make sure that babies or infants are placed in car seats properly when traveling by car. As the baby becomes more mobile emphasize the risk of falling or getting burned by hot surfaces.

- **Toddlers**

Toddlers are very curious, and they've already become fully mobile. Therefore, they are at an increased risk for accidents and injuries such as choking, drowning, poisoning, and more. Educate the parents and caregivers about the necessary safety precautions such as child-proofing the home. Also, talk about the importance of using car seats properly when traveling.

- **School-age children**

As the child grows, he becomes more and more independent, especially when he starts going to school and spending time with his friends. You can provide education to the children and their parents about traffic, water, and fire safety along with staying away from strangers. The law requires you to use car seats or boosters until the child weighs 80 lbs or reaches the height of 4'9".

- **Adolescents**

Those who are in this age group are at high risk because of their impulsivity, sense of being invincible, and their independence. You must provide education about motor vehicle safety both as a passenger and a driver along with the dangers of substance and alcohol abuse. It's also important to provide information about sexual health and safe sex practices.

- **Adults**

There are many kinds of risks for those in this age group in their workplace, home, and in other environments. Generally, you must review these risks with them, especially in terms of firearm use, motor vehicles, and fire safety.

- **Elderly adults**

Those in this age group may experience a decline in their cognitive and physical abilities which, in turn, increases their risks because of medications and of falls. They have a delay in their reaction times too which increases their risk of experiencing motor vehicle accidents. It's important to talk to patients in this age group as well as the people in charge of taking care of them.

No matter what the age of your patient is, you must familiarize yourself with the safety principles to prevent accidents relative to the care environment of your patients. These include:

- **Fall prevention program**

In healthcare facilities such as hospitals, falls are common among elderly adults and infants. You must know the different aspects of this program as well as the steps you need to take based on your patient's age.

- **Oxygen and suction equipment**

Make sure that your patient has access to oxygen and suction equipment. You must know when to use such equipment.

- **Seizure precautions**

For patients who are at risk for seizures, you must know how to keep them safe while they are seizing and after the episode.

- **Using restraints**

You may have to use restraints for patients who require a restriction of mobility because they have a high risk of seizures or falls. Also, this may be needed by patients who pose harm to other patients, other healthcare staff, and to themselves.

Infection Control

You must have a good understanding of infection control wherein you know all about the etiologic agent which is causing the infection. These pathogens may include fungi, bacteria, rickettsiae, helminths, protozoa, and others. Familiarizing yourself with how the infection spreads or the "chain of infection" is crucial for you to understand the precautions and interventions used to avoid it fully. To do this, you must know these elements:

- **Entry portals** which are the places where the infectious agents enter the susceptible hosts.

- **Exit portals** which are the places where the infectious agents leave their host.

- **Pathogens** which are the agents that cause the infection such as viruses or bacteria.

- **Reservoirs** which are the inanimate or animate environments which provide the pathogens with a favorable place for them to reproduce and grow.

- **Susceptible hosts** who are the patients or any other person who is at risk for getting an infection.

- **Transmission methods** which are the ways wherein the infectious organisms get transferred from the reservoirs to other susceptible hosts. The main transmission methods are airborne, indirect contact, and direct contact.

Preventing injuries, accidents or errors is heavily dependent on how well you can identify your patient's risk factors when he gets admitted to your healthcare facility. The developmental factors which we have already gone through along with the lifestyle of your patient and which safety precautions he is aware of will all be part of your assessment.

There are certain sensory deficits like

neuropathy, hearing, sight, proprioception, and more may all increase your patient's risk of accidents or injuries. One of the biggest issues which cause medical errors is medication allergies. Therefore, before you administer any type of medication to your patient, you must be prepared for an allergic reaction to the medication. In case any medical errors occur, make sure to follow the policies of your healthcare facility and think critically when making decisions.

Emergency Response Plan

The Joint Commission requires health facilities to have their plan for emergency responses. You may have to perform drills regularly to evaluate the efficacy of the emergency response plan of your healthcare facility. As a nurse, your responsibilities in the emergency response plan may differ depending on the healthcare facility. Most likely, you would have to ensure the safety of your patients first. Then you have to secure your facility by helping remove the threat of further danger or harm to your patients and the rest of the staff.

In case there is a fire, the first thing you need to do is to move your patients to a safe place.

Then, you may have to take the necessary steps to contain the danger (such as a fire) and lead your patients out of the building. Before doing this, you need to assess your patients to determine who can walk out of the hospital with some assistance and who needs to be brought out either in a stretcher or in a bed.

Ergonomic Principles

It's your responsibility to understand and make use of the correct ergonomic principles when you're helping your patients. This will prevent any injuries to yourself while still being able to help your patients function, ambulate, and avoid any injuries and accidents. You must incorporate these principles into your patient's care plan.

Assessing the baseline abilities of your patients will allow you to create an appropriate care plan which incorporates the utilization of various assistive devices like canes, walkers, and crutches. If you have a patient who has some form of repetitive stress injury, you must give him proper instructions about the proper body positioning which will help him avoid re-injury or the aggravation of his existing injury. For patients who have targeted conditions which only involve one muscular or skeletal group, you may provide them with instructions about proper stretching exercises and body positioning which will help reduce the stress felt on the affected area.

It's important to utilize the proper assistive devices and lifting techniques for patients as these will keep you and the other members of the healthcare facility from getting injured too. Your patient assessment, as well as your care plan, are crucial for the safety and protection of your patient and your safety, too. Also, you must know about and use the proper body positions and postures as you perform the daily functions at workstations which are technology-based such as mobile computers and desktops.

Hazardous Materials

Part of your responsibility is to properly and safely handle the equipment for patient care, potentially biohazardous or infectious materials, and any hazardous chemicals which are used in the healthcare facility. It's important for you to go through the Material Safety Data Sheets or MSDS. These are handouts which explain the potential hazards and nature and of the common chemical agents used in healthcare facilities. Familiarize yourself with the existence of these chemical agents and how to use them in case of an exposure. The Occupational Safety and Health Administration or OSHA mandates these.

Apart from the MSDS, the OSHA also came up with standards which they've written down and which discuss the standard precautions which you and everyone else in the healthcare facility must take to prevent exposure to blood-borne pathogens. It's important for you to know what you should do when a needlestick occurs, the environmental infection control standards, and the information associated with latex allergies for your patients and the rest of the healthcare staff.

Part of the written standards created by OSHA include the recommendations of the CDC for the proper use of the standard precautions. These refer to the standards for patient care which explain in detail how to keep the healthcare staff safe from blood-borne pathogens. Using PPE or personal protective equipment like face masks, eye protection, and gloves is essential whenever you encounter patients, especially in disaster or emergency response situations.

Apart from the different types of biohazardous materials, your workplace may also contain flammable materials as well as other potentially harmful substances. You must be aware of how to properly identify, store, and handle these materials. You must also know how to demonstrate safe practices safely to patients and the other members of the healthcare facility.

You must also be aware of the Needlestick Safety and Prevention Act which was implemented to protect the people who work in the healthcare setting. Safely disposing of any sharp materials must always be practiced along with the utilization of marked and mandated containers of biohazardous sharps in areas of patient care and preparation of medications. You must never recap used needles, and you must avoid breaking or bending them before disposing of them.

Home Safety

As a nurse, you play an important role in identifying, recommending, and implementing safety equipment and practices which are required by your patients in their home. Your patients and the members of their families would work with you throughout this process. The proper way to put home safety into practice is to teach your patients correct self-care methods and review any issues about children's safe care. The preventive measures for home safety also include the proper use of protective equipment when your patients utilize devices which are potentially dangerous at home.

Reporting Incidents

Throughout your career as a nurse, you're likely to be involved in writing incident reports. These reports are important tools which help you document all of the events which have led up to an accident and how you responded to it. It's important for you to learn the skills of reporting events both objectively and accurately when any unusual occurrence or incident happens. The overall goal of this activity is to avoid further injury or for the accident to happen again in the future. Each healthcare facility would have its guidelines to follow for the process of incident reporting. You must document all of the facts about the incident in your patient's medical records.

Equipment Use

Part of your responsibility is to endure the proper utilization and safety of all the equipment used in the care and treatment of patients. You may have to perform regular inspection and proper instruction to patients who need to make use of the equipment in their homes. If you discover that the equipment is either malfunctioning or is unsafe, you should stop using it, place a label to inform others that it's unsafe and place it somewhere where other healthcare staff can't access it for the care of patients. If possible, place the equipment in an area which has been specifically designated for malfunctioning or unsafe equipment and provide notice about the issue to the appropriate personnel.

Security Plan

In some cases, you may have to identify the patients who require urgent care in the event of an emergency or a natural disaster, and this is a very important task. To do this, you must perform a triage exam which has the purpose of identifying patients who require care to save their lives. This exam ensures that these patients are the first ones who receive proper assessment and treatment. It focuses on these areas:

- **Airway** wherein you must make sure that your patient's airway is open and clear.

- **Blood pressure** wherein you obtain your patient's blood pressure.

- **External bleeding** wherein you check for any indications of significant injuries or wounds in parts of the body which have major blood vessels.

- **Pulse** wherein you identify your patient's pulse then take note of its strength and rate.

- **Pupillary responses, state of the extremities, and consciousness** wherein you assess the neurological status of your patient, his consciousness level, how his pupils respond to light, paralysis symptoms or posturing the extremities.

- **Respiration** wherein you assess your patient for any indications of respiratory distress.

- **Respiration quality** wherein you assess your patient's breathing effort and rate then check for any indications of sufficient air exchange. Then auscultate your patients to listen to his breathing sounds.

You also play an important role in the event of bomb threats, lockdowns or security events in the newborn nursery, and evacuations of the healthcare facility. You may also be involved in the process of developing the emergency response plans for your healthcare facility. For these, you need to have critical thinking clinical decision-making skills for when you need to develop and implement these plans.

Precautions

There are several precautions used in the medical setting to prevent infections from spreading. The most common ones are the standard precautions which are utilized in all encounters with patients, precautions which are transmission-based which prevent pathogenic microorganisms from spreading, and the sterile technique or surgical asepsis which is utilized in surgical and other invasive procedures. Let's learn more about these precautions:

- **Standard precautions**

These include the utilization of PPEs such as gowns, masks, goggles, face shields, and more, which you must use when there is potential exposure to bodily fluids such as blood, excretions, and secretions. Using gloves and washing your hands are crucial precautions you must take to prevent the spread of infections and pathogens. When you use PPEs, begin by washing your hands outside of your patient's room. Then put on the gown, mask, goggles, and the gloves. When removing the PPEs, reverse the order and end with washing your hands.

- **Transmission-based precautions**

The spread of pathogenic microorganisms happens in different ways. You must know each of the specific transmission-based precautions (droplet, contact, and airborne) and when you should use each of these. In some cases, you may have to use more than one of these precautions. You must also familiarize yourself with the different infectious agents, how they are transmitted, and the specific precautions you need to take in the case of infections which are resistant to drugs.

- **Surgical Asepsis**

These precautions refer to the necessary practices which ensure that objects and areas are completely free from harmful microorganisms. Surgical asepsis is also known as the sterile technique, and it's used in surgical and other types of invasive procedures. Here are the basic principles to keep in mind:

- Each object utilized in a sterile field must also be sterile.

- If any of the sterile objects come in contact with an unsterile object, the objects are rendered unsterile.

- Any object which is below the level of the waist or is out of view is already considered unsterile.

- Any sterile object has the potential to become unsterile when it's exposed to airborne pathogens.

- Remember that all fluids flow in the direction of gravity.

- Fluids or moisture which

passes through a sterile object may draw pathogens from the unsterile surfaces below or above through capillary action.

- Any edges of sterile fields are considered unsterile.

- You cannot sterilize the skin.

Restraints and Safety Devices

These refer to tools which you can use to ensure the safety of your patients and the healthcare staff. Chemical restraints are medications while physical ones are jackets, bedside rails, and strap restraints for your patient's extremities. Familiarize yourself with how to use all of these, their indications, and the most effective and safe ways to use these restraints. It's important that you closely monitor your restrained patients frequently using different methods depending on what type of restraint you've used. Keep in mind that using restraints (no matter what type) comes with legal implications and you must familiarize yourself with these. Also, you must know all of the policies and procedures of your healthcare facility regarding restraints. Finally, you must also realize that there are specific medical conditions which often require the utilization of restraints.

Chapter 10: Taking the NCLEX-RN Exam

The NCLEX-RN differs from other exams in such a way that it determines whether or not you have the knowledge as well as the critical thinking skills needed to work as an entry-level nurse safely. We've just had a comprehensive look at the main categories to learn to prepare you for the exam. Now let's go through simpler but still relevant information which will help you out.

Try These Tested and Proven Study and Testing Tips

Now that you've studied the main categories which will appear on the NCLEX-RN, it's time to learn more about how you can effectively prepare for the actual test. Although this test can be very intimidating, preparing for it and trying your best to answer all of the questions to the best of your abilities can put your mind at ease. Here are some tested and proven tips for you as shared by registered nurses who have already passed the exam:

- Concentrate on your memorization and critical thinking skills.

- Prepare for the exam in advance and never cram for it.

- Apart from studying the concepts, study the exam as well.

- Take a lot of practice tests and answer a lot of practice questions during and after your review.

- When you're studying, spend more time on the concepts which you find difficult or those you had struggled with when you were still studying to become a nurse.

- When you go into the testing room, make sure that you are fully prepared to take the exam.

- While reading the questions, try to visualize the scenarios and think about what you would do if you were in them.

- While reading the answers, eliminate

those which you know are false first.

- Try not to stress yourself out before or during the exam.

- Speaking of stress, eliminate unnecessary stressors or sources of stress on the examination day.

- A few days before taking the exam, get a lot of rest.

- Dress comfortably and eat before taking the exam.

- Relax while you're taking the exam, so you don't lose your focus.

Avoid Test Preparation Burnout

Although preparing for the NCLEX-RN is very stressful for some people, it doesn't have to be. Don't stress yourself out in the preparation process or you might experience a burnout. When this happens, you will end up unmotivated and lacking the required confidence to do your best on the examination day. Here are some tips to help avoid test preparation burnout:

- **Make a plan**

Plans are important, so you don't feel overwhelmed with all of the information you need to learn for the exam. From learning about the test to learning the major categories, plan everything out, and you won't feel as overwhelmed or stressed about the whole process of preparation.

- **Study a bit each day**

Trying to study all of the concepts each day will surely burn you out. Instead, it would be better for you to set aside some time each day to prepare for the test. After that time, de-stress by doing activities which you enjoy. This will make you feel less stressed, and it will even make you feel more motivated to continue studying.

- **Incorporate exercise and a healthy diet into your plan**

Although these might not seem "related" with the test preparation, keeping yourself healthy will allow you to prepare better. If you feel good about yourself, the learning will come easier; thus, you will be able to review more efficiently.

- **Study in different ways**

There's nothing more monotonous and boring than simple reading text every day while trying to remember everything. To keep things interesting, study the concepts in different ways and different environments. That way, you will always have a fresh perspective each time you start studying. Doing this might even help you remember things better!

Mastering NCLEX-RN Style Questions

We've already gone through the different types of questions on the NCLEX-RN. Now let's go through some tips which may help you master the NCLEX-RN style questions:

- Identify **keywords** as these bear the most weight and are related to the patient, the problem, and the most important parts of the problem.

- Look for **repeated words** as this may help you select the correct answers.

- Look for **odd answers** which differ significantly from the other choices as this may be an indication for the right answer.

- Look for **opposite answers** as one of

those would usually be the correct answer.

- Consider the **"all of the above"** choice, especially when all of the answers seem to be applicable or correct.

- Eliminate the **incorrect answers**.

- Use the **prioritization technique** wherein all answers are correct so you must choose the one which takes priority over the others.

What to Bring on the Day of the Exam

After all of your studying and preparation, it's time for you to take the exam. On the exam day, there are specific items which you must bring. These include:

- **Documentation**

Before going into the testing room, you need to present your identification. Make sure to bring a government-issued ID which bears the exact name which appears on your ATT. Also, make sure your ID contains a photograph as well as your signature. You must also bring your ATT number which you will present at the testing center before they let you into the room.

- **Personal items**

You mustn't bring too many personal items to the testing center because you won't be allowed to take them with you inside the testing room anyway. You will be provided with a locker where you will keep your valuables including your watch, bag, coat, mobile phone, keys, and more. So only bring the essentials with you to ensure that everything fits in the locker.

- **Proper attire**

Although there's no dress code for taking the test, you should make sure to dress appropriately. Make sure that what you're wearing is comfortable enough, so you don't get distracted while you're taking the NCLEX.

- **Confidence**

This is one of the most important things to take with you, and the best part is, you are allowed to take this with you into the testing room! Leave your anxiety behind, relax, and take the test confidently. If you let your nerves get the best of you, this won't be productive. So think positively and do the best you can knowing that you've prepared for it.

Conclusion: Do Your Best When You Take the NCLEX-RN Exam!

The NCLEX-RN is the last hurdle you have to overcome before you can get your license as a registered nurse. This test is comprehensive, computer-adaptive, and is a requirement for all nursing graduates who want to work as registered nurses in Canada and the US. Therefore, you mustn't take it lightly if you plan to take it at all.

To prepare well for the NCLEX-RN, you need to familiarize yourself with it and learn everything that you can about it. There are different types of questions which you need to answer on this test, and we've discussed them all in the first chapter of this book. Of course, knowing the types of questions is just one aspect of the NCLEX-RN. Even though you have to answer different types of questions on this exam, there are some strategies which you can use to answer them including:

- **Don't read too much into the questions**

Take each of the questions at face value. Don't make assumptions about information which the question doesn't provide otherwise; you might choose the wrong answer. Focus on the question, and what it's asking so you can show that you're competent enough to care for your patients.

- **Think of the ideal situations**

The questions on the NCLEX-RN are based on an ideal world, one which most nurses can only hope for. Therefore, you must think of the ideal situations when choosing your answers rather than thinking about what you've learned in school or what you've experienced while working in a healthcare facility.

- **Consider the least invasive choices first**

Although some situations call for invasive procedures, it's better to choose the least invasive ones as long as they're reasonable.

- **The responses which are patient-focused are usually the correct ones**

Whenever you need to answer questions on the NCLEX-RN, you must always think about what's best for the patients. You will rarely find correct answers which will make your job easier than it is.

- **Search for clues which may hint at the correct answer**

Make sure to read the questions very well as some of them may contain clues which hint at the correct answers. Of course, don't look too hard. Sometimes these clues jump out at you when you least expect it.

- **Think about what the question is asking for**

When you're given situations, think about whether you need to perform an assessment or an intervention. This will make it easier for you to find the correct answer to those questions.

- **Consider the answers you must avoid**

Finally, there are certain answers which you must avoid when taking the NCLEX-RN. Always reconsider your answers, especially if they don't demonstrate action on your part. Generally, you should keep the following in mind:

- Never leave your patients, especially if they are unstable.

- Never choose to "do nothing," especially when it comes to patient care.

- Never pass the buck no matter how difficult the situation is.

- Only choose restraints as the last option, especially if there are other interventions you can do first.

- Never delay your patient's treatment.

With everything we've discussed and everything you've learned about the NCLEX-RN and what's on the NCLEX-RN, you are now ready to take the exam! As long as you remember and understand everything you've learned and you don't stress yourself out too much, you won't have to dread taking the exam. Good luck!

CPSIA information can be obtained
at www.ICGtesting.com
Printed in the USA
LVHW051305010621
689024LV00018B/1693